Occupational and Environmental Skin Disorders

Nlandu Roger Ngatu • Mitsunori Ikeda
Editors

Occupational and Environmental Skin Disorders

Epidemiology, Current Knowledge and Perspectives for Novel Therapies

Springer

Editors
Nlandu Roger Ngatu
Graduate School of Medicine
International University of Health
and Welfare (IUHW)
Chiba
Japan

Graduate School of Public Health
International University of Health
and Welfare (IUHW)
Tokyo
Japan

Mitsunori Ikeda
Graduate School of Nursing,
and Wellness and Longevity Center
University of Kochi
Kochi
Japan

ISBN 978-981-13-4231-8 ISBN 978-981-10-8758-5 (eBook)
https://doi.org/10.1007/978-981-10-8758-5

Printed on acid-free paper

This Springer imprint is published by the registered company Springer Nature Singapore Pte Ltd. part of Springer Nature
The registered company address is: 152 Beach Road, #21-01/04 Gateway East, Singapore 189721, Singapore

It has been almost 30 years since I was last treated by my mother for a skin disorder with the use of a plant-based remedy from her hometown in Congo. I knew this edible plant (V. amygdalina), given that its leaves were being used either as cough reliever or food in Africa. My first research projects as a Ph.D. candidate were related to experimental studies on animal models (and later on in human subjects) of eczematous disorders, skin conditions that are also induced by some factors found in the work and living environments. In recognition of their contribution to my current career as a researcher, I dedicate this work to my parents, Landu Pierre and Makiese Ngunda Berthe, and hope that many people, particularly those in rural Congo and Africa, will someday be relieved from common inflammatory skin disorders thanks to remedies from their rich nature. This work is also dedicated to my lovely wife, Yukimi Nakamura, for her wonderful support to my work, and to my son Kento-Landu Nakamura (Ken), of whom I am very proud for the progress he is making since he joined the university. I hope that, in near future, he will dedicate himself to serving humanity as a peace-loving scientist. Finally, this work is also dedicated to my parents-in-law, Masaru Nakamura and Yoshie Nakamura, for their wonderful support and care since I have been living in Japan.

Nlandu Roger Ngatu M.D., Ph.D.

Foreword

This book focuses on occupational and environmental skin diseases in terms of epidemiology, current knowledge, and perspectives for novel therapies. As the chairperson of the Allergy and Immunotoxicology Scientific Committee (SC) in the ICOH (International Commission on Occupational Health) and also the Vice-President of the Japanese Society for Hygiene (JSH), which aims to promote human health through integration of diverse factors associated with human life and the social and natural environment, it should be announced that this book is tremendously useful for researchers in the fields of occupational and environmental health as well as for regular citizens.

The skin is one of the gateways through which foreign bodies, biological and chemical agents enter the human body to cause conditions such as irritant, allergic, infectious skin disorders or cancers. It is almost permanently exposed to hazardous substances in the work and living environments.

This book covers several skin diseases caused by occupational and environmental hazards. The first part focuses on skin irritants, sensitizers, and carcinogens. Many novel chemical substances are developed and introduced in industrial work environments, and safety risk assessment of these newly developed hazardous substances is not vigorously performed. In particular, with respect to allergic substances, the relationship between human factors—such as sensitivities, HLA typing, and exposure frequencies and doses—and chemical characteristics is not considered uniformly according to the dose-response strategy.

Next, this book focuses on the environmental and occupational eczematous skin diseases, such as atopic and occupational contact dermatitis, with a particular consideration of risk factors, inflammatory mechanisms, pathophysiology, and therapeutic strategies, including steroids and nonsteroid agents. Since recent insights in molecular-targeting therapies for cancers and immune-related diseases such as autoimmune disorders have achieved better outcomes for various diseases, strategies to be employed for the treatment of allergic skin diseases should consider a detailed understanding of immune modulation that occurs in the course of these conditions.

The last part of this book includes environmental fungal, and also seasonal and endemic skin disorders caused by arthropods, insects, and microorganisms. I addition, it provides very informative highlights on silica dust-exposure and autoimmune diseases, particularly scleroderma. These are also very important, and a comprehensive understanding of these diseases may lead to a successful treatment and cure of people suffering from conditions resulting from the health effects of these environmental agents and associated infections internationally, especially in the developing world, including Africa, Asia, and Central and South America.

I am currently serving as chairperson of the Allergy and Immunotoxicology SC in the ICOH, which usually has a special session with the Occupational and Environmental Dermatoses SC, since these two SCs are closely related with investigating diseases and providing biological insights in allergy and immune responses. Recently, our SC published an eBook entitled *Allergy and Immunotoxicology in Occupational Health* in 2017 with Springer Nature publisher in the series "Current Topics in Environmental Health and Preventive Medicine" organized by the JSH. We recommend that people with an interest in "Occupational and Environmental Skin Diseases" read the aforementioned eBook to gain a better overall understanding and recognition of this field, the support required by patients with occupational and environmental skin diseases, as well as to develop preventive procedures. As an aside, there are various autoimmune diseases caused by occupational and environmental hazards, for example, systemic sclerosis is caused by silica, and vinyl chloride exposure. I hope another book that thoroughly explores cutaneous autoimmune diseases caused by occupational and environmental substances will also be planned by authors who contributed to this special book.

Finally, I strongly recommend researchers and other individuals who have an interest in occupational and environmental skin diseases to read this book and acquaint themselves with recent knowledge in these areas so that together we can overcome these diseases by being aware of their epidemiological, clinical and biological features, the use of novel therapeutics, as well as the development of preventive methods.

Kurashiki, Japan
January, 2018

Takemi Otsuki, M.D., Ph.D.

Preface

Occupational skin diseases (OSD) are prevalent work-related illnesses, ranking second after musculoskeletal disorders (MSD). The skin plays a crucial protective role mainly against numerous exogenous factors that threaten human health. Obviously, humans are constantly exposed to environmental and occupational pollutants that are part of the skin exposome. Yet, the human skin exposome has not yet received due attention (Krutmann et al. 2017) despite the overwhelming amount of hazards that jeopardize people's health both at home and at the workplace. The growing industrialization and the rapid urbanizations of cities and towns generate a wide variety of health hazards, bringing tremendous changes in the living and working environments. Air pollution, which is identified as a global health priority in the WHO's sustainable development goals (SDGs), affects human health; and several studies have shown striking results in terms of the negative effects of environmental pollutants on skin health. For example, children living in areas with higher traffic-related air pollution have been reported to have higher risk of developing allergic disorders. Additionally, studies on the relationship between ambient air pollutants (particulate matter, oxides, ozone, cigarette smoke) and skin health have shown that environmental pollutants trigger and aggravate atopic dermatitis (Yi et al. 2017). Furthermore, several other substances present in occupational settings and/or in the general environment (metals, dusts, fibers, chemicals) are associated with OSD.

The present work includes an overview of occupational skin hazards and approaches for their assessment, original contributions (based on a Ph.D. thesis, both experimental and clinical studies), and reviews on topics related to occupational and environmental eczematous disorders, common environmental dermatomycoses and other seasonal and epidemic skin diseases, their epidemiology, risk factors, clinical features, as well as preventive and therapeutic approaches. The text, which provides updated knowledge and insights on those conditions, is a product of an interdisciplinary work and was written by a group of scientists who have been working together for years. One particularity of this work is that it mainly explores, in a single volume, most common and prevalent occupational and environmental skin disorders that specialists and researchers in the field often meet in their practice. Our hope is that readers will gain insights into current knowledge on skin conditions described in this book and ways to prevent and manage them.

Chiba, Japan
Kinshasa, D.R. Congo

Nlandu Roger Ngatu, M.D., Ph.D.

References

Krutmann J, Bouloc A, Sore G, et al. The skin aging exposome. J Dermatol Sci. 2017;85(3):152–61.

Yi SJ, Shon C, Min KD, et al. Association between exposure to traffic-related air pollution and prevalence of allergic diseases in children, Seoul, Korea. Biomed Res Int. 2017;2017:4216107.

Acknowledgments

To those who have been supporting us in the process of writing this book and those who gave us useful advice, our research collaborators, at Kochi University Medical School and the University of Kochi in Japan, at the Faculty of Medicine of the University of Kinshasa and William Booth University in the Democratic Republic of the Congo, we are very thankful to them:

Professor Suganuma Narufumi, Dean of Kochi University Medical School and Chief of the Department of Environmental Medicine, who mentored one of the editors (NRN), for his continued support;

Professor Nojima Sayumi, President of the University of Kochi, Japan, for supporting our work and provided us with a good environment for conducting research projects;

Professor Longo-Mbenza Benjamin, scientist and lecturer at the Facutly of Medicine of the University of Kinshasa and University President Kasa-Vubu, Democratic Republic of the Congo, for his rich advice;

Dr. Saruta Takao, Director of Saruta Dermatological Clinic in Kochi prefecture, Japan, for his wonderful support to this work;

Dr. Kalubi Bukasa Jean-Baptiste, Associate Professor at the School of Medicine of Osaka University, for his advice and guidance;

Finally, we are also thankful to colleagues and research collaborators for their support: Professor Andre Renzaho, at the School of Social Sciences and Psychology, Western Sydney University, Australia, and Dr. Muchanga Sifa Marie-Joelle, researcher at the National Center for Global Health and Medicine, Japan, and the Department of Gynecology and Obstetrics, Faculty of Medicine, University of Kinshasa, Democratic Republic of the Congo.

Nlandu Roger Ngatu, M.D., Ph.D.
Mitsunori Ikeda, M.D., Ph.D.

Contents

1 **Introduction** 1
Nlandu Roger Ngatu

Part I Skin Irritants, Sensitizers and Carcinogens

2 **Skin Function and Occupational Skin Hazards** 7
Nlandu Roger Ngatu

Part II Environmental and Occupational Eczematous Skin Disorders

3 **Atopic Dermatitis (or Atopic Eczema)** 23
Nlandu Roger Ngatu and Mitsunori Ikeda

4 **Occupational Contact Dermatitis** 41
Nlandu Roger Ngatu

5 **Quality of Work Environment and Frequency of Work-Related Dermatitis Among Dust-Exposed African Informal Coltan Miners** 53
Ngombe Leon-Kabamba, Nlandu Roger Ngatu, Etongola Papy Mbelambela, Melaku Haile Likka, Sakatolo Jean-Baptiste Kakoma, Numbi Oscar Luboya, Roger Wumba, and Brigitta Danuser

6 **Occupational Cement Dermatitis and Cement Burns** 63
Ngombe Leon-Kabamba, Sakatolo Jean-Baptiste Kakoma, Numbi Oscar-Luboya, Mukanya Pascal-Kimba, Nkulu C. Banza-Lubamba, Nlandu Roger Ngatu, and Benoit Nemery

7 **Alternative Nonsteroidal Therapies for Occupational and Environmental Allergic Skin Disorders** 71
Mitsunori Ikeda

8 Sacran: Novel Sulfated Polysaccharide as Anti-Allergic Skincare Biomaterial for Atopic Dermatitis 79
Keiichi Motoyama, Taishi Higashi, Nlandu Roger Ngatu, Maiko Kaneko Okajima, Yasumitsu Nishimura, Hidetoshi Arima, and Tatsuo Kaneko

9 Clinical Anti-Allergic Effects of African *Vernonia amygdalina* Leaf Extracts 93
Nlandu Roger Ngatu

10 Experimental Anti-Allergic and Immunomodulatory Effects of *Vernonia amygdalina*-Derived Biomaterials, Vernodalin and Its Leaf Extracts 105
Ryoji Hirota and Nlandu Roger Ngatu

Part III Fungal, Neglected Seasonal, Epidemic and Other Environmental Kin Disorders

11 Common Environmental Dermatomycoses 119
Nlandu Roger Ngatu

12 Sarcoptic Skin Disease (or Scabies) 133
Roger Wumba and Nlandu Roger Ngatu

13 Frequency and Clinical Features of Sarcoptic Skin Disease (Scabies) in Congolese Schoolchildren 143
Roger Wumba and Nlandu Roger Ngatu

14 Paederus Dermatitis: Environmental Risk Factors, Clinical Features, and Management 151
Nlandu Roger Ngatu

15 Overview on Other Environmental Skin Disorders 159
Nlandu Roger Ngatu and Mitsunori Ikeda

Contributors

Hidetoshi Arima, Ph.D. Graduate School of Pharmaceutical Sciences, Kumamoto University, Kumamoto, Japan

Brigitta Danuser, M.D., Ph.D. Service of Occupational Medicine, Institute for Work and Health, University of Lausanne and Geneva, Epalinges-Lausanne, Switzerland

Etongola Papy Mbelambela, M.D., M.Sc. Department of Environmental Medicine, Kochi Medical School, Kochi University, Kochi, Japan

Taishi Higashi, Ph.D. Graduate School of Pharmaceutical Sciences, Kumamoto University, Kumamoto, Japan

Ryoji Hirota, Ph.D. Department of Nutrition, Matsumoto University, Nagano, Japan

Mitsunori Ikeda, M.D., Ph.D. Graduate School of Nursing, and Wellness & Longevity Center, University of Kochi, Kochi, Japan

Maiko Kaneko Okajima, Ph.D. School of Materials Science, Japan Advanced Institute of Science and Technology (JAIST), Nomi, Japan

Tatsuo Kaneko, Ph.D. Polymer Science, Energy & Environment, Japan Advanced Institute of Science and Technology (JAIST), Nomi, Japan

Melaku Haile Likka, B.Sc., M.P.H./H.S.M. Health informatics, Department of Health Information Science, Kochi Medical School, Kochi University, Kochi, Japan

Pascal Kimba Mukanya, M.D., M.P.H. Toxicology, Unit of Toxicology and Environment, School of Public Health, University of Lubumbashi, Lubumbashi, Congo

Benoit Nemery, M.D., M.P.H. Occupational & Environmental Medicine, Department of Public Health and Primary Care, KU Leuven, Leuven, Belgium

Leon-Kabamba Ngombe, M.D., M.P.H. Toxicology, Unit of Toxicology & Environment, Department of Public Health, Faculty of Medicine, University of Kamina, Kamina, Congo

Yasumitsu Nishimura, Ph.D. Immunology & Gerontology, Department of Hygiene, Kawasaki Medical School, Kurashiki, Japan

Celestin Banza-Lubamba Nkulu, M.D., Ph.D. Toxicology, Unit of Toxicology and Environment, School of Public Health, University of Lubumbashi, Lubumbashi, Congo

Oscar Luboya Numbi, M.D., Ph.D. Public Health & Pediatrics, School of Public Health and Faculty of Medicine, University of Lubumbashi, Lubumbashi, Congo

Faculty of Medicine, University of Kamina, Kamina, Congo

Stanislas Wembonyama Okitotsho, M.D. Ph.D. Public Health & Pediatrics, School of Public Health & Faculty of Medicine, University of Lubumbashi, Lubumbashi, Congo

Nlandu Roger Ngatu, M.D., Ph.D. Graduate School of Medicine, International University of Health and Welfare (IUHW), Chiba, Japan

Graduate School of Public Health, International University of Health and Welfare (IUHW), Tokyo, Japan

Jean-Baptiste Kakoma Sakatolo, M.D., M.M.ed., Ph.D., A.E.S.M. Public Health & Parasitology, School of Public Health & Faculty of Medicine, University of Lubumbashi, Lubumbashi, Congo

School of Public Health & School of Medicine, College of Medicine & Health Sciences, University of Rwanda, Kigali, Rwanda

Roger Wumba, M.D., Ph.D. Faculty of Medicine, University William Booth, Kinshasa, Congo

Parasitology & Molecular Biology, Department of Tropical Medicine, Faculty of Medicine, University of Kinshasa, Kinshasa, Congo

Chapter 1
Introduction

Nlandu Roger Ngatu

Abstract Advances in industrialization have contributed to environmental pollution, which represents a major risk to the health of populations. On the other hand, increased incidence of skin diseases has been reported both in developed and developing countries due to high levels of hazardous substances in the working and living environments; these include physical, animal, and chemical particulates. This book provides updated knowledge and information on the epidemiology, etiology, and physiopathology of prevalent occupational and environmental skin diseases (OESD), their prevention, with particular emphasis on skin health safety issues and disease risk factors present at workplace and in the living environment, as well as recent progress on their management. It comprises a PhD thesis and original reports, perspectives and review articles as well. Thus, it can be useful for occupational and environmental health practitioners, academic lecturers, researchers, graduate students, and clinicians in the field of skin diseases. Recent studies have shown that the prevalence of allergic diseases, for example, increased sharply in many rich countries; however, their management is still challenging due mainly to the limitation in treatment choices and the adverse effects related to most of the existing conventional therapeutic agents. At workplace, the establishment of a safety and health service, organizing a surveillance and reporting systems for dermal exposures at workplace, and a strict compliance with safety measures and occupational exposure limits for skin hazards (for chemical hazards particularly), as well as the implementation of efficient and affordable therapeutic procedures for OESD, are of utmost importance.

Keywords Exposure · Occupational and environmental skin disease (OESD) · Prevention · Skin hazard

N. R. Ngatu, M.D., Ph.D. (✉)
Graduate School of Medicine, International University of Health and Welfare (IUHW), Chiba, Japan

Graduate School of Public Health, International University of Health and Welfare (IUHW), Tokyo, Japan

N. R. Ngatu, M. Ikeda (eds.), *Occupational and Environmental Skin Disorders*,
https://doi.org/10.1007/978-981-10-8758-5_1

List of Abbreviations

ESD	Environmental skin diseases
NIEHS	National Institute of Environmental Health Sciences
NIOSH	National Institute for Occupational Safety and Health
OESD	Occupational and environmental skin diseases
OSD	Occupational skin diseases

1.1 Progress in Technology, Industrialization, and Scope of Skin Disorders in Occupational Settings

Recent advances in industrialization have contributed to environmental pollution, a major risk to the health of populations worldwide. High levels of hazardous substances at workplace and in the living environment are reported to have increased the incidence of skin disorders both in developed and developing countries. The indoor and outdoor pollution involve exposures to physical agents, animal, mineral, and chemical particulates that may directly threaten human health, particularly through skin contact or their penetration into the respiratory tract (NIEHS 2017). According to a recent report from the US National Institute of Occupational Health and Safety (NIOSH), an estimated 13,000,000 workers in the USA are subject to exposure to chemicals that can be absorbed through the skin (NIOSH 2013).

Occupational and environmental skin diseases (OESD) comprise cutaneous disorders that are caused or triggered by occupational or environmental hazards. If occupational skin diseases (OSD) are disorders of the skin that are caused by or worsened by exposures to hazards at workplace (EU-OSHA 2008), on the other hand, ESD are disorders of the skin that are caused by exposure to environmental hazards. OSD are reported to be one of top three registered occupational diseases in the European continent (HSE 2016), and they are costly, with an estimated 600,000,000 EUR spent annually and 3,000,000 lost working days (EU-OSHA 2008). In the USA, OSD are the most commonly reported non-traumatic occupational health diseases. Given their negative impact on workers' vocational and avocational activities, OSD have a considerable socioeconomic impact (Lushniak 2003), suggesting their public health importance. In the 1990s, OSD represented 13% of all occupationally acquired diseases in the USA; and the US Bureau of Labor Statistics has estimated the annual cost associated with OSD to reach one billion dollars (NIOSH 1996).

1.2 Objectives of This Book

This book provides updated knowledge on the epidemiology, etiology, and pathophysiology of several prevalent OSD and ESD, with a particular emphasis on skin health safety issues, risk factors, preventive measures, and recent progress on their management. It also highlights recent discoveries and developments on novel therapeutic agents for occupational and environmental skin inflammatory disorders, especially findings that are supported by clinical data. We hope that this work will be useful to occupational and environmental health researchers, lecturers, as well as clinicians and medical graduate students.

1.3 Skin Exposure, Risk Management, and Perspectives for Efficient Risk Control

Nowadays, almost everyone is daily subject to dermal exposure to occupational and/or environmental hazards, particularly chemical agents that may affect the skin health. Thus, changes in the work or living environment should be monitored and be addressed using appropriate interventions aimed at preventing their potential health consequences. Considering occupational and environmental health approach for the diagnosis and management of work-related ailments, which aims at caring not only for the sickened individuals but the group or even the exposed population, there is a necessity to initiate strategies for effective health risk assessment and identification, disease prevention among exposed groups and populations, and disease management and control.

Recent studies have suggested that the prevalence of allergic skin disorders has sharply increased in industrialized countries in the past few decades (Romagnani 2004), atopic dermatitis in particular. However, the management of these skin disorders remains challenging due mainly to the limitation in treatment choices. In several countries, steroids are still the unique remedy; in order to prevent the occurrence of side effects in susceptible individuals or manage skin lesions located at body areas where steroids are not indicated, alternatives to steroidal drugs are already in use. Additionally, environmental changes have brought up new cutaneous hazards that contribute to the increase of a number of environmental skin disorders whose management is somewhat challenging suggesting the necessity of novel therapeutic options.

Obviously, workplace skin exposure assessment is scarcely implemented in occupational settings compared to inhalation exposures (NIOSH 2013), and the situation is alarming in most developing countries where work safety still remains a neglected concept. It is also evident and unequivocal that the diagnosis of occupational skin diseases is very challenging, particularly for health professionals not specialized in the field, given that the involvement of factors present in the work environment is not thought of in most clinical settings. Another reason is about follow-up challenges, as some patients visiting the hospitals for skin disorders never return to see their doctors; this makes difficult the implementation of further etiologic investigations that could lead to the identification of the occupational origin of the disease. Furthermore, when the involvement of an occupational hazard is considered, its identification may necessitate hard work, requiring the implementation of risk assessment procedures that would eventually lead to the determination of the cause of disease. In addition, the establishment of an occupational safety and health service, the organization of a surveillance and reporting systems for dermal exposures at workplace (where skin health risks exist), and a strict compliance with safety measures and occupational exposure limits for skin chemical hazards at work settings, as well as the implementation of effective and affordable therapeutic procedures for diagnosed OSD cases, are of utmost importance.

References

European Agency for Safety and Health (EU-OSHA). Skin diseases and dermal exposure: policy and practice overview. 2008. osha.europa.eu/en/publications/factsheets/40/view. Accessed 1 Sep 2017.

Health & Safety Executive (HSE). Statistics: dermatitis and other skin disorders. 2016. http://www.hse.gov.uk/statistics/causdis/. Accessed 1 Sep 2017.

Lushniak BD. The importance of occupational skin diseases in Unites States. Int Arch Occup Environ Health. 2003;76(5):325–30.

National Institute of Environmental Health Sciences (NIEHS). Air pollution. 2017. https://www.niehs.nih.gov/health/topics/agents/air-pollution/index.cfm. Accessed 1 Sep 2017.

National Institute of Occupational Health and Safety (NIOSH). Disease and injury. 1996. https://www.cdc.gov/niosh/docs/96-115/diseas.html. Accessed 1 Sep 2017.

National Institute of Occupational Health and Safety (NIOSH). Skin exposures and effects. 2013. https://www.cdc.gov/niosh/topics/skin/default.html. Accessed 1 Sep 2017.

Romagnani S. The increased prevalence of allergy and the hygiene hypothesis: missing immune deviation, reduced immune suppression, or both? Immunology. 2004;112(3):352–63.

Part I
Skin Irritants, Sensitizers and Carcinogens

Chapter 2
Skin Function and Occupational Skin Hazards

Nlandu Roger Ngatu

Abstract Human skin is the largest organ, representing 15% of body weight and serving as external protective barrier for the entire body. The skin has important physiological functions that are vital for the organism, such as the protective role, the thermoregulatory function, waterproofing, tactile sensation, and the synthesis of vitamin D. On the other hand, the skin can also serve as the site of passage for hazardous substances such as chemicals that threaten human's health, given that it is exposed to environmental and occupational hazards that may cause injury, skin sensitization, irritation, or systemic disorders. A number of occupations are known to expose workers to skin sensitizers and irritants (medical professionals, dental technicians, construction workers, farmers, florists, hairdressers, estheticians, metal workers, mechanics, machinists, miners, printers, textile workers, etc.), whereas others are subject to contact with skin carcinogens (road construction workers, coal gas manufacturers and handlers, pitch loaders, brick and tile workers, timber proofers, cutting oil and lubricant manufacturers and handlers, aluminum reduction workers, oil refinery workers, insecticide manufacturers and handlers, paraffin wax workers, etc.). To promote occupational safety and health of workers, implementing periodic educational sessions and training to increase awareness on the health risks posed by hazards at workplace and performing biological monitoring in the work environment with sampling workstations and the skin are among the safety measures for hazard assessment and risk control.

Keywords Risk assessment · Risk control · Skin carcinogen · Skin hazard · Skin irritant · Skin sensitizer

---

N. R. Ngatu, M.D., Ph.D.
Graduate School of Medicine, International University of Health and Welfare (IUHW), Chiba, Japan

Graduate School of Public Health, International University of Health and Welfare (IUHW), Tokyo, Japan

N. R. Ngatu, M. Ikeda (eds.), *Occupational and Environmental Skin Disorders*,
https://doi.org/10.1007/978-981-10-8758-5_2

Abbreviations

EASHW	European Agency for Safety and Health at Work
HRA	Health risk assessment
ICMM	International Council on Mining and Metals
OEL	Occupational exposure limit
OSH	Occupational safety and health
PPE	Personal protective equipment
RCAP	Risk control action plan

2.1 Overview on the Anatomy and Physiology of the Skin

The skin is the largest organ of human body, representing approximately 15% of body weight (Kolarsick et al. 2011). It comprises three layers (Fig. 2.1):

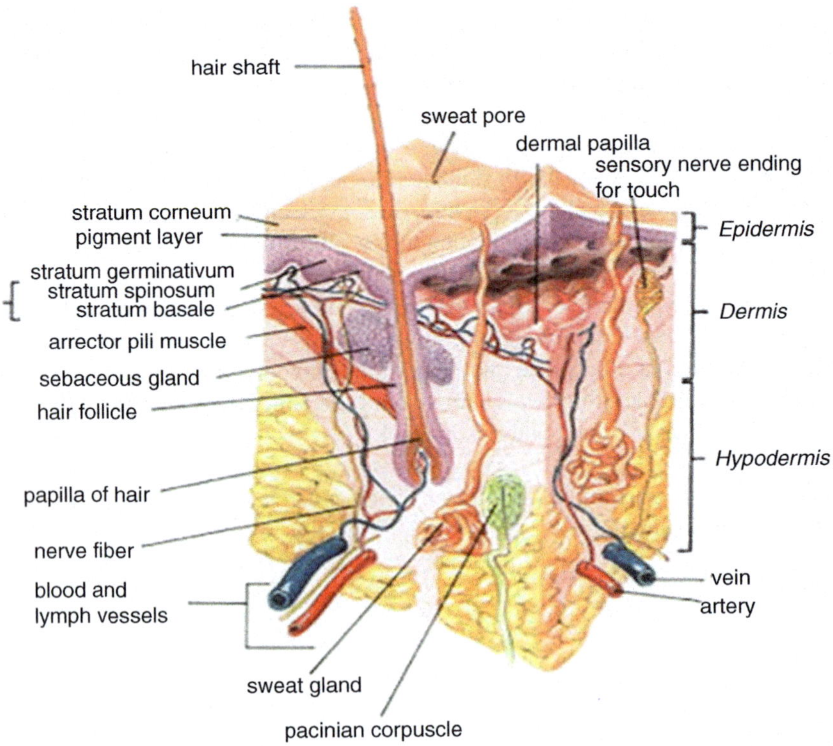

Fig. 2.1 Skin anatomy. The figure shows layers of the skin and anatomical components of the cutaneous tissue (Hill 2017). [© Dr. Mark Hill 2017, UNSW Embryology ISBN: 978 0 7334 2609 4-UNSW CRICOS Provider Code No. 00098G (image unmodified)]

1. *Epidermis*: it consists of a constellation of cells called keratinocytes that produce keratin, a protein with a protective role. This layer has no blood vessels; thus it is dependent on the underlying middle layer (dermis) for its nutrient delivery and also for waste disposal through the dermo-epidermal junction. The epidermis itself has layers: the *stratum germinativum* or basal layer, *stratum spinosum*, *stratum granulosum*, and *stratum corneum*. The epidermis comprises four types of cells:
    - *Keratinocytes*: they divide and differentiate, moving from deeper layer to superficial ones. In the *stratum corneum*, keratinocytes are fully differentiated and lack nuclei.
    - *Melanocytes:* they can be found in the basal layer of the epidermis, in hair follicles, in the eye's retina, and in leptomeninges; their primary function is to produce melanin, a pigment that absorbs radiant energy from the sun and protects the skin from the harmful effects of UV radiation. Melanocytes are the sites of origin for melanoma.
    - *Langerhans cells:* originating from bone marrow, they are found in basal, spinous, and granular layers of the epidermis, serving as antigen-presenting cells.
    - *Merkel cells:* they are present on the volar aspect of digits, in nails, and other areas of the skin; they are specialized in the perception of light touch.
2. *Dermis*: it is the middle layer made up of a fibrillary structural protein known as collagen; its function is to support and sustain the epidermis. It comprises two layers: the papillary dermis (which is more superficial) and the deeper one, the reticular dermis (thicker layer of dense connective tissue that contains larger blood vessels, fibroblasts that produce procollagen, mast cells, nerve endings, lymphatics, and epidermal appendages).
3. *Subcutaneous tissue*: it contains small lobes of fat cells called adipocytes.

The thickness of each of the skin layers varies according to geographic location on the body. For example, the eyelid has the thinnest epidermis that measures less than 0.1 mm, whereas the palms and soles of the feet have the thickest epidermis layer, measuring about 1.5 mm. The middle layer or dermis is thicker on the back (Kanitakis 2002; Burns et al. 2004; Berger & Elston 2006).

The skin has several vital function that includes the following:

1. Protection against external physical, chemical, and biological agents
2. Thermoregulation and prevention of excess water loss from the body
3. Shock absorption (thanks to its elasticity) and waterproofing (the skin barrier prevents not only the penetration of water but also other environmental agents)
4. Tactile sensation (sensory organs are present in the skin allowing humans to recognize tactile stimuli and others)
5. Synthesis of vitamin D (Kanitakis 2002)

Apart from those physiological functions that are beneficial for humans, the skin can serve as the passage for hazardous substances such as chemicals that threaten human's health. In addition, the skin is also exposed to environmental and occupational agents that either cause an injury (abrasion, contusion, laceration), induce cutaneous reaction that will manifest in the form of inflammation, or cause chemical poisoning (e.g., toxicant substances) after their absorption through the skin. Cutaneous absorption of toxicants is tributary to a number of factors, such as:

- Skin integrity at the time of exposure to the hazard
- Location of exposure
- Duration of exposure
- Surface area of exposed skin
- Physical and chemical properties of the hazard (NIOSH 1999)

2.2 Chemical Skin Hazards in Occupational Settings

The International Labor Office (Birmingham 2011) provides a list of sectors and industrial settings with potential exposure to skin health hazards. For example, workers exposed to chromates, epoxy and phenolic resins, thinner, glues, turpentine (construction workers), latex rubber, local anesthetics, disinfectants, detergents, alcohol (healthcare professionals), nickel, gold, formaldehyde, glutaraldehyde, eugenol (dentists), insecticides, plants (farmers, florists, gardeners), paraphenylenediamine in hair dye, perfume, oils, preservatives in cosmetics, surfactants in shampoos, bleach, acetone, peroxide (hairdressers, estheticians), metals, abrasives (miners, metal workers, mechanics, machinists), color developers, acrylic monomer, and amine catalysts (printers, photographers) may develop skin allergic reaction or irritation (Table 2.1).

On the other hand, a number of agents found in several occupational as well as nonoccupational settings are currently known to cause skin cancer. For example, exposure to pitch-black resin (tar and tarry products) at work, for example, at aluminum reduction station in coal, gas, or coke industries or in the environment, can cause cutaneous cancer. Pitch (resin) is known as viscoelastic polymer of natural origin (plant material) or manufactured. Bitumen and asphalt are forms of pitch; this material has also been used for shipbuilding and to make waterproof wooden containers and torches (The Netherlands 2008). A report from the International Agency for Research on Cancer (IARC) that is based on a cohort study has concluded that sufficient evidence was found in regard to the carcinogenicity of coal-tar on human skin. The study has reported more than 700 cases of skin cancers caused by occupational exposures during coal-tar distillation, suggesting an increased risk of cutaneous cancer among coal-tar exposed workers (Brownstein and Rabinowitz 1979; IARC 2010). Other occupations at risk are briquette makers, road construction workers, brick and tile workers, as well as timber proofers.

Table 2.2 presents a list of chemical substances that are most incriminated in the development of occupational skin cancer. Since the middle of the twentieth century, the relationship between coal-tar and tarry products and skin disorders has been

Table 2.1 Common chemical sensitizers, irritants, and corresponding occupations

Occupations	Irritants	Sensitizers
Construction workers	Turpentine, thinner, glues, fiberglass	Chromates, epoxy and phenolic resins, colophony, turpentine, woods
Dental technicians	Detergents, disinfectants	Rubber, epoxy and acrylic monomer, formaldehyde, glutaraldehyde amine, catalysts, anesthetics, mercury, gold, nickel, eugenol
Farmers, gardeners, and florists	Detergents and soaps, fertilizers, disinfectants	Plants, woods, insecticides, fungicides
Food handlers, cooks, bakers	Detergents/soaps, vinegar, vegetables, fruits	Benzoyl peroxide, spices, garlic, vegetables, rubber
Hairdressers, estheticians	Shampoos, bleach, peroxide, acetone	Paraphenylenediamine in hair dye, ammonium persulfate in bleach, surfactants in shampoos, nickel, perfume, essential oils, preservatives in cosmetics, glyceryl monothioglycolate in permanents
Medical professionals	Disinfectants, soaps and detergents, alcohol	Colophony, formaldehyde, latex (rubber), antibiotics, anesthetics, phenothiazines, benzodiazepines, glutaraldehyde, disinfectants
Metal workers, mechanics, machinists, miners	Detergents and soaps, cutting oils, petroleum distillates, abrasives	Biocides in cutting oils, nickel, cobalt, chrome, epoxy resins and amine catalysts, hydrazine and colophony in welding flux, rubber
Printers and photographers	Solvents, acetic acid, ink, acrylic monomer	Nickel, cobalt, chrome, rubber, formaldehyde, paraphenylenediamine, azo dyes, hydroquinone, epoxy and acrylic monomer, amine catalysts, color developers
Textile workers	Solvents, bleaches, natural and synthetic fibers	Formaldehyde resins, azo- and anthraquinone dyes, rubber, biocides

Table 2.1 shows nonexhaustive list of common occupational irritants and sensitizers (Birmingham 2011; NISOH 2012a)

established. A report by Ross (1948) suggested that tar and pitch cause eczematous reaction, acanthosis, keratosis, telangiectasia, and, at later stages, cutaneous squamous cell carcinoma. Soot (made of carbon resulting from incomplete hydrocarbon combustion in chimney sweeps), cutting oils and lubricants (cotton industry, glass blowing stations, paraffin wax processing, oil refining industries, automatic machine shops), and arsenic (chemical in the environment and insecticides used by farmers and gardeners, oil refinery stations, etc.) are other known skin carcinogens (Table 2.2). Another study conducted among employees of a tar refinery showed that exposure to this health hazard induced an increased incidence of new cases and relapse of malignant skin tumors in exposed employee population (Voelter-Mahlknecht et al. 2007). The authors have suggested the necessity to intensify preventive measures not only for the workers but also the general public with evident exposure to tar and tarry products.

Table 2.2 Skin cancer-associated substances and occupations at risk

Skin carcinogenic agent	Industry/hazard	Process/group at risk
Coal-tar pitch, tarry product	Aluminum reduction	Pot room workers
	Coal, gas, and coke industries	Coke ovens, tar distillation, coal gas manufacture, pitch loading
	Patent fuel manufacture	Briquette making
	Asphalt industry	Road construction
	Creosote users	Brick and tile workers, timber proofers
Soot	Chimney sweeps	
Lubricating and cutting oils	Glass blowing	
	Shale oil refining	
	Cotton industry	Mule spinners
	Paraffin wax workers	
	Engineering	Tool setters and setter operators in automatic machine shops (cutting oils)
Arsenic	Oil refinery	Still cleaners
	Sheep dip factories	
	Arsenical insecticides	Manufacturing workers and users (gardeners, fruit farmers, and vintagers)

Table 2.2 shows information of skin carcinogens and related occupations (Birmingham 2011)

Metal-working fluids (MWFs) such as lubricants and cutting oils are commonly used in machinery and grinding operations in numerous industrial settings. Despite their usefulness in cooling and extending the life of machines and grinders, they also represent a risk to the health of exposed workers. Millions of workers are daily exposed to these hazards. Several reports have shown that MWFs cause skin cancers, as well as respiratory disorders in exposed populations (Jarvholm et al. 1981; Jarvholm et al. 1985; IARC 1987; Kennedy et al. 1989; Li et al. 2003).

The cutaneous toxicity of arsenic (As) and arsenic compounds (both inorganic and organic chemicals) has been well established both in several animal experiments and clinical studies. As is a metalloid or semimetal chemical belonging to group VA of the periodic table, and it is one of the most common element in the earth's crust. Its presence in the environment is a result of volcanic eruption and industrial activities, which contaminate the air, water, and soil (WHO 2001); thus, humans in general, and workers in particular, can be exposed to arsenic or its products through inhalation, ingestion, or direct contact to the skin. This suggests the importance of assessment of arsenic-related health risk in the work environment, as well as in the living environment where the risk of contamination or intoxication is evident. Three major groups of arsenic compounds are toxic for the skin:

1. *Inorganic arsenic compounds* (arsanilic acid [$C_6H_8AsNO_3$], metallic arsenic [As], arsenic oxide [As_2O_3; As_2O_5], arsenic sulfide [As_2S_3], arsenic chloride [$AsCl_3$], arsonium [$C_5H_{11}AsO_2$]): their current and historical uses include

pharmaceuticals (leukemia, psoriasis, and bronchial asthma treatment), wood preservatives, agricultural chemicals (pesticides, insecticides, herbicides, soil sterilants, defoliants, etc.), applications in mining, glassmaking, metallurgical manufacturing, and semiconductor industries (IARC 2017).

2. *Organic arsenic compounds* (calcium arsenate or arsenic acid, cacodylic acid, lead arsenate, methanearsonic acid, potassium arsenite, potassium arsenate, sodium arsenate, sodium arsenite, sodium cacodylate) (IARC 2017): they are also used as agricultural pesticides. The US Environmental Protection Agency has canceled their use and ordered their elimination in 2009 (EPA 2009); exception was made for monosodium methanearsonate (MSMA).
3. *Arsine gas*: also known as arsenic hydride, it is a toxic substance that is generated from other arsenic compounds by some bacteria and fungi species. On the other hand, an unintentional formation of arsine occurs mainly in metallurgical industries as a result of arsenic contamination of zinc, lead, copper, cadmium, antimony, silver, tin, or gold during contact between these arsenic-bearing ores and acid. Workers are exposed to toxic levels of arsine during processes such as electrolytic refining, galvanizing, lead plating, metal smelting, and extraction (Suess et al. 1985; WHO 2001, 2017). Arsine's toxicity is established for the nervous system, liver, and kidney, and it causes hemolysis. However, its carcinogenicity remains controversial. A report from the New Jersey Department of Health (2008) suggests that arsine is carcinogenic and can cause skin and eye damage in case of direct contact.

2.3 Assessment and Management of Cutaneous Chemical Hazards: First Step Toward OESD Prevention

Chemical hazards in occupational settings have to be assessed for their identification and their toxicity. In occupational settings, work safety staff should design plans that combine information on existing health hazards and instructions that workers should observe in order to protect the workers and prevent hazard-related disorders. For example, skin care and cleaning products should be available at workstations where exposure to skin hazards is either possible or evident. With the cooperation of the employers, periodic educational sessions and training to increase workers' awareness on the health risks posed by the chemical hazards, in addition to biological monitoring in the work environment, with sampling of workstations and the skin, should be performed to ensure hazard assessment and risk control.

According to the US-based National Institute for Occupational Safety and Health (NIOSH), occupational risk assessment consists of estimating health risks from exposure to various levels of a hazard at workplace (NIOSH 2017). And the purpose of health risk assessment (HRA) is to find answers to the below questions:

- What can happen (in the presence of the hazard)?
- How likely is it to happen?
- And what are the health consequences in case it happens?

On the other hand, the International Council on Mining and Metals (ICMM) considers occupational HRA as a process involving the following four elements:

1. Identification of hazardous substances and their sources
2. Estimation of the potential for exposure and related health effects
3. Quantification of exposures
4. Assessment of the risks through the use of appropriate techniques and the identification and assessment of control measures' effectiveness (ICMM 2015)

Unlike the purely clinical approach common to most medical disciplines that are mainly oriented toward disease diagnosis and treatment at health settings, occupational safety and health (OSH) specialists would primarily focus on the identification and management of the risks to the health of workers and, eventually, the community members living in the surrounding environment, mostly prior to disease occurrence or just after a case is diagnosed. It is worth it, given that the occurrence of even a single case of occupational disease caused by a health risk present in the work environment indicates a failure to protect the health of the workers, and that reducing the level of risk or eliminating it to avoid the appearance of another case is considered a more reasonable approach in OSH and would ensure the safety and health of the workforce (ICMM 2015; The Netherlands 2008). Below, we summarized the steps required for occupational and environmental health risk assessment, as shown in Table 2.3.

Table 2.3 General approach to health risk assessment (HRA) in 13 steps

1	**Identification of HR and their sources** at work environment and associated health effects
2	**Identification of potentially exposed individuals** (workers, local residents)
3	**Identification of processes, tasks, and areas of occurrence of hazardous exposures**
4	**Assessment, measurement, or verification of the exposures**
5	**Assessment of potential health risks posed by the hazardous exposures**, for example, exposure duration, frequency of exposure, level of exposure versus occupational exposure limit (OEL), etc.
6	**Rating and prioritizing health risks** (high, medium, low)
7	**Identification of existing control measures and assessment of their effectiveness**
8	Establishment of **risk and control measures register**
9	Deciding on **risk acceptability** and setting **priorities for action**
10	Implementation of corrective action—**development, implementation, and monitoring of a risk control action plan (RCAP)**—or reviewing existing RCAP
11	**Timely reinstatement of control measures if they fail**
12	**Maintaining accurate and systematic records of HR** or amend existing RCAP; use alternative and/or additional control measures
13	**Reviewing and amending implemented interventions** at regular intervals or earlier if new development are proposed

HRA health risk assessment, *HR* health risk, *ICMM* International Council on Mining and Metals, *OEL* occupational exposure limit, *RCAP* risk control action plan. The table contains risk assessment steps as proposed by ICMM (2015)

The progress of technology surely brings up a lot of advantages to the people, as it facilitates access to their needs such as improved communication tools, mass production of easily affordable food products, low-cost food and energy, transportation, etc. However, it also comes with new hazards that populations have to face in their work or living environment. Therefore, while being eager to benefit from these new technologies, health professionals and policy makers should be concerned to identifying health risks associated to them, with anticipation. Hence, there is always a need to carry out investigations designed to find out environmental or workplace health risks, determine exposure limits, and propose safety measures to be implemented so as to mitigate the exposure and avoid any nuisance that the new hazards might cause. This suggests the importance of risk assessment and monitoring, a first and important step in promoting occupational safety and health at workplace. Failing to identify the health risks is exposing workers and, sometimes, the local population to health issues or accidents that might be of unpredictable magnitude or even catastrophic.

Hazards to skin health are numerous in several occupational and environmental settings. However, less initiatives have been taken to ensure the safety of workers against skin hazards in settings with mechanical, physical, chemical, or biological agents with potential to cause accident or harm the skin. In Fig. 2.2, we summarized the framework of HRA for hazard identification and characterization in the work and living environment.

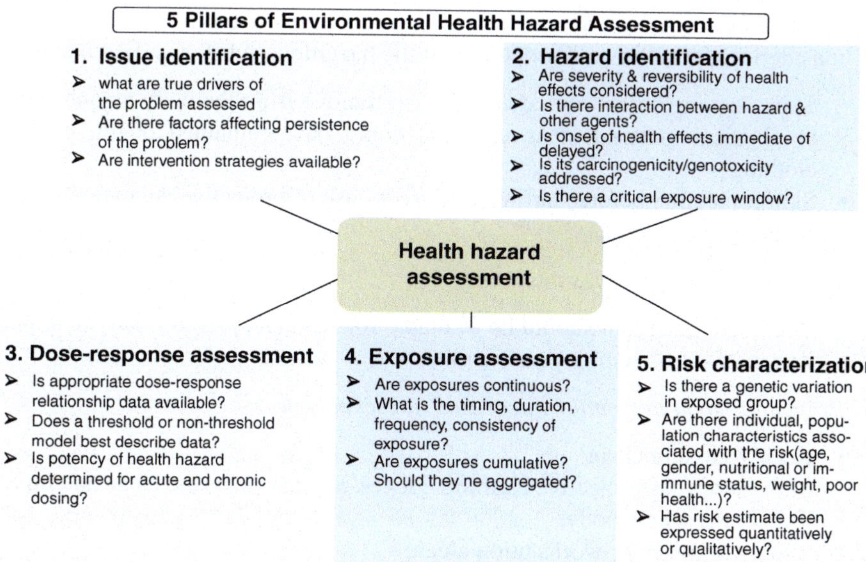

Fig. 2.2 Framework of health risk assessment process for hazard identification and characterization. (Diagram produced by authors based on Guidelines of the Department of Health, Australia 2012)

2.4 Strategic Framework for Exposure Prevention to Skin Hazards in Occupational and Environmental Settings

To prevent exposure to skin hazards and related cutaneous disorders, different occupational health organizations have proposed main interventions to be implemented at workplace. The Australian Department of Health (2012) has recommended the following:

1. *Engineering control of the hazard:* it consists of interventions aimed at eliminating the hazardous substance and its substitution or replacement. When the elimination of the health hazard is not envisaged, a number of measures can be used to control the exposure and reduce the risk, such as the use of ventilation systems, the development of processes that can minimize workers' exposure to the hazard, designing or redesigning the equipment or tool, and source capture or source modification to limit the spread of the contaminant in the air.
2. *Use of alternatives to hand manipulation:* providing suitable and effective personal protective equipment (PPE) to workers. Most of the time, this option is much less costly than engineering control. Use of adapted gloves, clothing, and other garments that protect workers from a contact with hazardous substances at work settings can markedly reduce exposure. However, safety staff should make sure that the PPE used by workers does not have a potential to cause harm to the workers' health (latex rubber, leather, and other sensitizing and irritant materials should be avoided).
3. *Drawing up skin protection plan*: this may include a number of measures and instructions susceptible to promote work safety at occupational settings while considering the nature and properties of the hazardous substance. For example:
   - Skin cleaning before and after work (to remove from the body any chemical or physical material, dust, etc. that could have remained on the skin or clothing)
   - Skin protection before starting work (e.g., use of protective device)
   - Skin care after work
4. *Making washing facilities available*
   - Water and detergent should be available for workers, preferentially at a location not far from employees' workstation
5. *Promoting good personal hygiene and housekeeping*
   - Keep your skin clean.
   - Make sure your protective clothing, gloves, and garments are clean and intact.
   - Protect the whole body.
   - Keep workplace or workstation clean.

In addition to what is said above, in order to protect the workers and prevent the occurrence of occupational skin disorders, the NIOSH has proposed simplified *hierarchy control measures* employers should undertake that we summarized below

Table 2.4 Skin health risk control measures (based on NIOSH recommendations for OSD prevention at workplace (2012b)

Action for skin health risk control	Importance and meaning
1. Elimination of skin health hazard	Most effective control method to prevent skin damage or contact with hazardous chemical or product
2. Substitution of the skin hazard	Hazardous or harmful chemical or product can be replaced by a less harmful one to reduce the risk of skin disease
3. Engineering control	When the harmful product cannot be eliminated or substituted for any reason, another intervention should be envisaged to reduce the risk, for example, the use of exhaust ventilation systems or use of isolation booths to avoid skin contact with the hazard
4. Administrative control	Organization of "work safety training programs" to educate workers on hazards at workplace and how they should protect themselves from those hazards
5. Personal protective equipment (PPE)	Use of devices or equipment that prevent direct contact of the skin with the hazard, for example, safety glasses or goggles, appropriate gloves, shop coats, coveralls, boots, etc., to prevent exposure to glue, epoxy resins, detergents, disinfectants, solvents, other cleaning products and chemicals, etc.

(Table 2.4). To summarize, at the workplace or in the living environment, when a substance or product that represents a skin health hazard is identified, it should be eliminated and, eventually, be replaced (substitution) by a safer or less harmful product. However, when for any reason the elimination and the substitution are not envisaged, the hazardous substance or product can be modified (engineering control) to reduce the risk of disease or injury.

Another measure often implemented in occupational settings with skin health risk is to have employers and occupational safety and health specialists organize periodic education and training for workers to increase awareness on the health risks presented by the hazards and provide knowledge and skills on how to protect themselves (administrative risk control). One of the preventive measures used to control skin health hazards is the use of personal protective equipment (PPE). Furthermore, in any occupational setting, a timely reporting of any skin disorder that might be associated with exposure to a hazard at work should be a rule; and medical screening should be undertaken to identify other workers having the same health issue and preventive measures implemented to prevent the occurrence of other cases.

References

Berger JWD, Elston TG. Andrews diseases of the skin: clinical dermatology. 10th ed. Philadelphia: Elsevier Saunders; 2006.

Birmingham DJ. Skin disease. International Labor Office (ILO) encyclopedia of occupational health and safety. 2011. http://iloencyclopaedia.org/part-i-47946/skin-diseases/23-12-skin-diseases/overview-occupational-skin-diseases. Accessed 22 Sep 2017.

Brownstein MH, Rabinowitz AD. The precursors of cutaneous squamous cell carcinoma. Int J Dermatol. 1979;18(1):1–16.

Burns DA, Breathnach SM, Cox N, Griffiths CE, editors. Rook's textbook of dermatology. 7th ed. Malden, MA: Blackwell Science; 2004.

Department of Health (Australia). Environmental health risk assessment: guidelines for assessing human health risks from environmental hazards, 2012. http://www.health.gov.au/internet/main/publishing.nsf/content/health-pubhlth-publicat-environ.htm.

Environmental Protection Agency (EPA). Organic arsenicals; product cancellation order and amendments to terminate uses. 2009. https://www3.epa.gov/pesticides/chem_search/reg_actions/reregistration/frn_UG-5_30-Sep-2009.pdf. Accessed 11 Oct 2017.

Hill M. Embryology: skin structure cartoon. 2017. https://embryology.med.unsw.edu.au/embryology/index.php/File:Skin_structure_cartoon.jpg. Accessed 22 Dec 2017.

International Agency for Research on Cancer (IARC). Mineral oils (lubricant based oils and derived products). In Volume 33. Polynuclear aromatic hydrocarbons, Part 2, carbon blacks, mineral oils (lubricant based oils and derived products) and some nitroarenes. Lyon, France: IARC Scientific Publications; 1987. p. 87–168.

International Agency for Research on Cancer (IARC). Occupational exposures during coal-tar distillation (IARC report 2010). 2010. https://monographs.iarc.fr/ENG/Monographs/vol100F/mono100F-16.pdf. Accessed 2 Oct 2017.

International Agency for Research on Cancer (IARC). Arsenic and arsenic compounds (IARC report 2017). 2017. http://monographs.iarc.fr/ENG/Monographs/vol100C/mono100C-6.pdf. Accessed 11 Oct 2017.

International Council on Mining and Metals (ICMM). Good practice guidance on occupational health risk assessment. 2nd ed. 2015. https://www.icmm.com/website/publications/pdfs/health-and-safety/161212_health-and-safety_health-risk-assessment_2nd-edition.pdf. Accessed 12 Sep 2017.

Jarvholm B, Lillienburg L, Sallsten G, et al. Cancer morbidity among men exposed to oil mist in the metal industry. J Occup Med. 1981;23:333–7.

Jarvholm B, Fast K, Lavenius B, et al. Exposure to cutting oils and its relation to skin tumors and premalignant skin lesions on the hands and forearms. Scand J Work Environ Health. 1985;11:365–9.

Kanitakis J. Anatomy histology and immunohistochemistry of normal human skin. Eur J Dermatol. 2002;12(4):390–401.

Kennedy SM, Greaves LA, Kriebel D, et al. Acute pulmonary responses among automobile workers exposed to aerosols of machining fluids. Am J Ind Med. 1989;15:627–41.

Kolarsick P, Kolarsick M, Goodwin C. Anatomy and physiology of the skin. J Dermatol Nurses Assoc. 2011;3(4):203–13.

Li K, Aghazadeh F, Hatipkarasulu S, Ray TG. Health risks from exposure to metal-working fluids in machining and grinding operations. Int J Occup Saf Ergon. 2003;9(1):75–95.

National Institute for Occupational Safety and Health (NIOSH). Occupational risk assessment. 1999. https://www.cdc.gov/niosh/topics/riskassessment/default.html.

National Institute for Occupational Safety and Health (NIOSH). Skin exposures and effects (NIOSH 2012). 2012a. https://www.cdc.gov/niosh/topics/skin/default.html.

National Institute for Occupational Safety and Health (NIOSH). Skin exposures and effects: recommendations and resources. 2012b. https://www.cdc.gov/niosh/topics/skin/recommendations.html.

National Institute of Occupational Health and Safety (NIOSH). Disease and injury. 2017. https://www.cdc.gov/niosh/docs/96-115/diseas.html. Accessed 1 Sep 2017.

New Jersey Department of Health. Arsine: hazardous substance fact sheet. 2008. http://www.nj.gov/health/eoh/rtkweb/documents/fs/0163.pdf. Accessed 11 Oct 2017.

Ross P. Occupational skin lesions due to pitch and tar. Br Med J. 1948;2:369–74. https://www.ncbi.nlm.nih.gov/pmc/articles/PMC2091422/pdf/brmedj03691-0013.pdf

Suess MJ, Grefen K, Reinisch DW. Ambient air pollutants from industrial sources. Amsterdam: Elsevier; 1985. pp 419, 420, 457, 458
The Netherlands. Coal-tar pitch, high temperature; summary risk assessment report, 2008. https://echa.europa.eu/documents/10162/13630/trd_rar_env_netherlands_pitch_en.pdf. Accessed 2 Oct 2017.
Voelter-Mahlknecht S, Scheriau R, Zwahr G, et al. Skin tumors among employees of a tar refinery: the current data and their implications. Int Arch Occup Environ Health. 2007;80(6):485–95.
World Health Organization (WHO). Arsenic and arsenic compounds; WHO report 2001. 2001. http://apps.who.int/iris/bitstream/10665/42366/1/WHO_EHC_224.pdf. Accessed 11 Oct 2017.
World Health Organization (WHO). Arsine: human health aspects. 2017. http://www.who.int/ipcs/publications/cicad/en/cicad47.pdf. Accessed 11 Oct 2017.

Part II
Environmental and Occupational Eczematous Skin Disorders

Chapter 3
Atopic Dermatitis (or Atopic Eczema)

Nlandu Roger Ngatu and Mitsunori Ikeda

Abstract Atopic dermatitis (AD) is a chronic relapsing, and severely pruritic skin disorder. AD is considered one of the major public health problems in the world, and its prevalence is increasing, especially in industrialized countries. This report contains updated knowledge on AD, its epidemiology, and current diagnostic and management approaches. There are approximately 10–20% of children and 1–3% of adult population affected worldwide. According to the International Study of Asthma and Allergies in Childhood (ISAAC), AD is most prevalent in developed and westernized countries. In most western countries, AD diagnosis is made by considering a number of clinical features (Fig. 3.1) and patient's history, classified into two categories, major and minor criteria, a system developed by Hanifin and Rajka in the 1980s. Sometimes, AD diagnosis is challenging, given the similarities in clinical features with other conditions. The disease severity is estimated using a number of scoring systems, of whom SCORAD is the most commonly used. It takes into account the intensity of each of the five AD skin lesions (redness, swelling, oozing/crusting, scratch marks, lichenification), in addition to pruritus (itch) and sleeplessness, and also the area of affected body parts. With the rising AD incidence and its familial association, new prophylactic strategies are being investigated. Currently, emollient and probiotic preparations provide a new hope in AD prevention in individuals at risk. Bacterial (*Staphylococcus aureus*) and viral (*herpes simplex*) infections are the most prevalent in complications. These complications may justify the use of anti-allergic agent combined with an antibiotic or antiviral drug in some AD patients, in addition to conventional anti-allergic drugs. Finally, most commonly used conventional AD treatment agents are presented in this work.

Keywords Atopic dermatitis · Cytokine · Filaggrin · Skin barrier

---

N. R. Ngatu, M.D., Ph.D. (✉)
Graduate School of Medicine, International University of Health and Welfare (IUHW), Chiba, Japan

Graduate School of Public Health, International University of Health and Welfare (IUHW), Tokyo, Japan

M. Ikeda, M.D., Ph.D.
Graduate School of Nursing, and Wellness & Longevity Center, University of Kochi, Kochi, Japan

N. R. Ngatu, M. Ikeda (eds.), *Occupational and Environmental Skin Disorders*,
https://doi.org/10.1007/978-981-10-8758-5_3

Abbreviations

AD Atopic dermatitis
FLG Filaggrin
GM-CSF Granulocyte-macrophage colony-stimulating factor
IFN-γ Interferon gamma
IgE Immunoglobulin E
IL Interleukin
NMF Natural moisturizing factor
TGF-1β Transforming growth factor 1 beta
Th T-helper
TNF-α Tumor necrosis factor alpha
TSLP Thymic stromal lymphopoietin

3.1 Introduction: Definition and Epidemiology of Atopic Dermatitis

Atopic dermatitis (AD) or atopic eczema is a chronic relapsing and severely pruritic allergic skin disorder (Darsow et al. 2005; Williams 2005; Furue et al. 2017). The disease is also characterized by redness and scratch markings (Fig. 3.1). The prevalence of AD is increasing, especially in industrialized countries. AD is considered as one of the major public health problems in the world; it is a disease whose expression and development are influenced by genetic and environmental factors (Sehgal et al. 2015). Approximately, 10–20% of children in the world are affected by AD (Lee et al. 2006; Leung 2000; Kawakami et al. 2007), whereas 1–3% of adult population are affected worldwide (Nutten 2015).

According to the International Study of Asthma and Allergies in Childhood (ISAAC) which involved two million children in 100 countries of the world, AD is most prevalent in developed and westernized countries and least prevalent in the most non-westernized and underdeveloped countries. In Norway, for example, cross-sectional prevalence of AD in children from 7 to 13 years of age is reported to

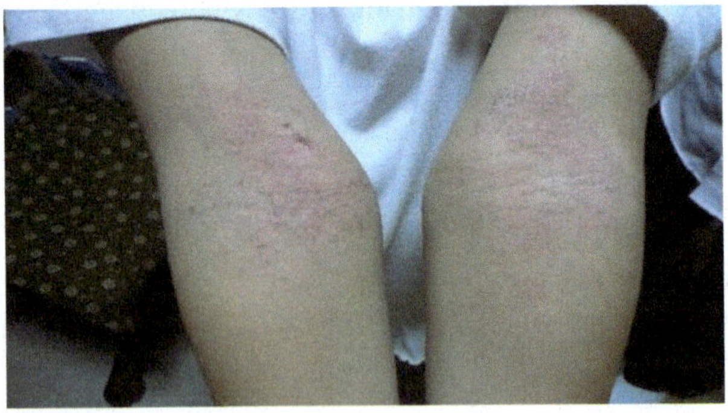

Fig. 3.1 Atopic dermatitis skin lesions (erythema, papules, and scratch markings) on left and right arms of an 11-year-old girl who was taken care of during a preliminary clinical trial (Ngatu et al. 2015)

be 19.7%. In England, the point prevalence in 3–11-year-old children is reported to be 1.5–14%. Furthermore, recent reports showed that, for children aged between 6–7 years, prevalence of 0.9% in India and 22.5% in Ecuador were found; on the other hand, 0.2% in China, 24.6% in Columbia, and over 15% in Africa, Latin America, and Europe (Nutten 2015).

Japan is one of the countries with high AD prevalence rate. However, rates depend on cities, with most industrialized sites being most affected. Additionally, proportions of 9.5% and 20% have been reported on the Japanese archipelago (Benn et al. 2004). In the United States, allergic contact dermatitis is one of the most prevalent work-related illnesses and has been estimated to cost billion US dollars annually (Diepgen and Blettner 1998). A cross-sectional survey conducted in Kinshasa, Democratic Republic of Congo (DRC), by Nyembue et al. (2011) showed that, of the 1326 participants with rhinitis who underwent skin prick test (SPT), 31.6% were sensitive to common local aeroallergens, suggesting a relatively high proportion of the Congolese population from Kinshasa could be atopic with AD predisposition.

3.2 Risk Factors and Pathogenesis of Atopic Dermatitis

Investigations on AD pathogenesis have previously been focusing primarily on generalized immune system abnormalities in T-helper 1 and T-helper 2 (Th-1/Th-2) activity. However, recently, research has been shifting to more targeted immunologic abnormalities and the impairment of the barrier function (Sullivan and Silverberg 2017). It is likely that there are two groups of AD patients, with one group experiencing skin barrier defect as the *primum mobile* in AD development and then induces abnormalities of the immune system, and another group in which immunologic abnormalities occur first and later on cause the impairment of the barrier function. Understanding those complex phenomena that trigger the development of AD will allow new research approaches that target different pathways related to allergic inflammation induction in AD, thus making the finding of novel potent and suitable therapies for different AD phenotypes.

3.2.1 Genetic Factors Associated with Atopic Dermatitis

AD is an allergic disease with a complex genetic background, showing a strong maternal influence. A family history of AD is obtained in about 70% of patients. Clinically normal parents may have affected children, excluding a simple dominant inheritance; whereas, in other families, both parents may be affected by the disease but the children are normal, excluding a simple recessive trait. A number of population-based surveys have shown that the risk of developing AD in children was higher when the mother was atopic than when the father was and that the transmission of AD and other atopic disorders occurs frequently through mothers (Ruiz et al. 1992; Sehgal et al. 2015).

Immunoglobulin E (IgE) and Th-2 cytokines play an important role in the pathogenesis of AD, and genes involving those inflammatory mediators have been identified, for example, susceptibility loci on 1q21, 3p24–22, 3q21, and 17q2 are associated with AD. Additionally, several other loci associated with AD severity and IgE (e.g., 3q14, 3p26–24, 4p15–14, 13q14, 15q14–15, 17q21, 18q1–12, 18q21, 18q20) were found (Williams et al. 1999; Sehgal et al. 2015; Kwan and Burrows 2009). Moreover, genes on chromosome 5q encoding the cytokine gene cluster have also been associated to atopic mucosal syndrome as well as polymorphism in the interleukin-4 (IL-4) gene with AD, and another gene at 16p11.2–12 that encodes the chain of IL-4 receptor has also been linked to atopic status (Doull et al. 1996; Oiso et al. 2000). Furthermore, variants of RANTES gene promoter region have been linked to AD (Nickel et al. 2000), and a polymorphism in the gene encoding high-affinity IgE receptor FCR1 chain has been reported to have a strong association with AD (Sandford et al. 1993).

It has been reported that increased total serum IgE and specific IgE antibody to the allergen is the main immunological abnormality in AD. Approximately 80% of AD patients are thought to have higher total IgE levels; this suggests that the more severe and extended the disease becomes, the more the level of total serum IgE increases (Champion et al. 1998; Blumenthal and Amos 1998).

3.2.2 *Role of Environmental Factors*

Several previously published works have suggested that the current increased AD prevalence cannot be explained solely by genetic changes in the population. Thus, it has been suggested that environmental factors such as pollution and also microbes play a role as contributing factors. Cohorts of preschool children from comparable cities in Germany that took into account socioeconomic status, history of AD, and the monitoring of airborne pollutants have shown lower AD prevalence in rural than urban population (Schafer et al. 1996; Yemaneberhan et al. 2004).

Other reports have suggested that, in individuals with the atopic phenotype, eczema may be induced or exacerbated by either staphylococcal toxins or the presence of Malassezia yeasts on the skin. Thus, the role of microbes in the early maturation of the immune system could be the major factor that may explain differences between the western world and the developing countries in regard to the incidence of atopy and allergic diseases such as AD (Strachan 2000).

Regarding microbial role, a number of individual factors linked to exposure to microbes that can protect against or increase AD severity have recently been proposed. For example, dog exposure in early life and day-care attendance in the first 2 years of life may play a protective role, whereas postnatal antibiotic and high endotoxin exposure levels during the first year of life are considered as risk factors for AD (Nutten 2015).

Furthermore, a recent work by Kim (2015) suggested that the estimated lifetime prevalence of AD has increased two to three fold during the past 30 years particularly in urban areas in industrialized countries. The report attributes this fact to the increased exposure to various environmental chemicals such as air pollutants (e.g., benzene, PM2.5, PM10, nitrogen oxide compounds, and CO exposure), skin irritants, contact allergens, food additives, and ingredients in cosmetics, rather than the alterations in human genome. Air pollutants from combustion of engines, industrial factories, and heating systems in buildings have been associated with a greater prevalence of allergic diseases in industrialized countries. In addition, a number of epidemiological studies have suggested that some of the air pollutants were responsible for the development or the exacerbation of AD and other allergic disorders (Montnemery et al. 2003; Pénard-Morand et al. 2010; Song et al. 2011; Kim et al. 2013).

A recent study by Japanese researchers has provided a new understanding on the role of air pollution in triggering the development of cutaneous allergic inflammation in atopic individuals (Hidaka et al. 2017) have discovered a receptor (aryl hydrocarbon receptor, AhR) that links AD to air pollution via the induction of the neurotrophic factor artemin (ARTN). AhR activation by air pollutants induced expression of artemin, alloknesis, epidermal hyper-innervation, and inflammation which positively correlated in the epidermis of AD patients. Thus, environmental stimuli are sensed by keratinocyte's AhR that elicits the allergic reaction (AD).

Controlling exposure to environmental factors that increase AD risk would contribute to reducing the incidence of this skin condition. Of the risk factors that trigger the development of AD, a report by Nutten (2015) has recently proposed the following:

- Pollution and tobacco smoke
- Low outdoor temperature
- Intake of fast food
- Delayed weaning
- Obesity

On the other hand, a number of measures are susceptible to exert protective effect against AD. Their promotion might help to reduce AD prevalence in children population particularly. They include (nonexhaustive list):

- Intake of fresh fruits
- Fish intake (by the mother during pregnancy)
- UV light exposure
- Breastfeeding

In fact, studies have shown that breastfeeding beyond 3 months of age has a protective effect on the infant and that, for those of infants who cannot be breastfed, prolonged feeding with a partially hydrolyzed whey formula may result in a 45% reduction in infantile AD among at-risk infants (Alexander and Cabana 2010; Szajewska and Horvath 2010; Nutten 2015).

3.2.3 Novel Insight: Role of Filaggrin (FLG) Mutation

Although FLG mutation alone may not account for the pathogenesis of AD, its role in the disease pathogenesis has been established (Seguchi and Cui 1996; Brown and McLean 2012; Newell et al. 2013; Ong 2014). Of the group of proteins that make the skin barrier, FLG is believed to be the most important as it contributes to the formation of natural moisturizing factor (NMF) (Irvine et al. 2011). The skin barrier prevents water loss from the skin and the intrusion by microorganisms and skin irritants (Brown and McLean 2012). It has been reported that 26.7% of AD children have decreased expression of FLG. However, apart from FLG defect, recent investigations have suggested that other skin barrier genes are likely to account for barrier defects in AD patients without FLG (Morar et al. 2007; Marenholz et al. 2011), for example, abnormalities of lipid composition, excessive serine protease activity which is caused by mutations in SPINK5 gene encoding for lymphoepithelial Kazal-type-related inhibitor (Elias and Steinhoff 2008), claudins of tight junction, or the suppression of skin barrier by the inflammation (De Benetto et al. 2011; Ong 2014).

3.2.4 Immune Deviation Toward Th-2 and Th-22 Expansion

In atopic individuals, lesional AD skin exhibits Th-2 (IL-4, IL-5, IL-13) and T22 (IL-22)-deviated immune reactions in the acute phase of the disease. Then, it progresses toward chronicity, a phase in which Th-1 cytokine (IFN-γ)-expressing cells are predominant. This Th-2/Th-1 shift can also be observed in atopic patch test elicited by house dust mite antigen (Furue and Kadono 2015; Furue et al. 2017). Atopic status is associated with preferential activation of Th-2 phenotype CD4 T cells; these cells produce IL-4 and IL-5 which stimulate IgE synthesis by B cells. On the other hand, the production of Th-1 cytokines such as interferon gamma (IFN-γ) is reduced in AD, indicating a fundamental cytokine dysfunction (Coleman et al. 1993).

A report by Tesmer et al. (2008) explained the sequential T-helper cell involvement in AD. After the first contact with the allergen or other factors such as microbes (mostly *Staphylococcus aureus*), the antigen-presenting cells will migrate to regional lymph nodes where they will present processed peptides to naïve T cells. Then, the latter will differentiate, in the presence of the inflammatory marker IL-4, and induce the production of IgE by B lymphocytes. A consecutive binding circulating IgE to high-affinity IgE receptors on tissue-resident mast cells will then occur. During a second exposure to the same allergen, a cell reactivation will be induced along with mast cell degranulation and the consecutive release of inflammatory molecules such as histamine, IL-8, and IL-13, creating an environment that will cause an influx of Th-2 lymphocytes and eosinophils into the skin, leading to the production of Th-2 cytokines such as IL-4, IL-5, and IL-13. Those Th-2 cytokines will, in turn, stimulate eosinophils to release IL-25. The Th-2 environment will then be enhanced in this acute phase of the disease (AD).

Furthermore, the stimulation of eosinophils will also induce the release of IL-6, IL-1, and transforming growth factor 1 beta (TGF-1β) which in turn supports Th-17 cells' differentiation and recruitment to the skin where they interact with Th-2 cells, keratinocytes, and fibroblasts. Additionally, to IL-6, IL-1, and TGF-1b, eosinophils (epidermal and dermal dendritic cells as well) will also produce IL-12 which will activate Th-1 cells to produce Th-1 cytokines (IFN-γ) driving the shift to the chronic phase (Tesmer et al. 2008).

Other recent researches proposed the importance of the role played by interleukin-22 (IL-22)-producing T (T22) cells and Il-17-producing Th-17 cells in the initiation and the maintenance of allergic inflammation in AD patients, in addition to CD3+ T cells, CD11c + dendritic cells, and CD1c + dendritic cell infiltrations in the acute phase of AD and more intensely in the chronic phase of the disease (Gittler et al. 2012; Furue et al. 2017). Nogratesand colleagues were the first to demonstrate T22 cell accumulation in lesional skin of AD. Those T22 cell infiltrates include CD4+ helper (Th-22) and CD8+ cytotoxic (Tc22) cells; of the two, only Tc22 cells are correlated to the clinical severity of AD (Nograteset al. 2009). Moreover, Gittler and colleagues have found an upregulation of genes related to Th-2 (IL-4, IL-10, IL-31, CCL11) and T22 (IL-22, S10A7, S100A8, S100A9, S100A12, IL-32) in AD skin lesions during the acute phase. This fact is further associated with an upregulation of Th-1-related genes (IFN-γ, CXCL9, CXCL10, and CXCL11) in the chronic phase of AD (Gittler et al. 2012). In addition, a concomitant increase of chemokine receptors (CCL1, CCL4, CCL13, CCL17, CCL18, CCL20, CCL22, CCL26, CXCL1, CXCL2, CXCL3, CXCL8, CXCL10, CCR1, CCR7) and enhanced expression of Janus kinases (JAK) 1 and 3 (Gittler et al. 2012; Czamowicki et al. 2015; Sugaya et al. 2015; Esaki et al. 2016) are reported to occur in the course of atopic inflammation.

3.2.5 *Role of Keratinocytes in Immune Dysfunction in AD*

Located in the *stratum corneum* of the epidermis, keratinocytes are epithelial cells that are primary cellular source of the skin barrier deficiency in AD. In AD patients, keratinocytes have an increased expression of granulocyte-macrophage colony-stimulating factor (GM-CSF), tumor necrosis factor alpha (TNF-α), and thymic stromal lymphopoietin (TSLP), a pro-Th-2 IL-17 cytokine. Mascia et al. (2010) have found that GM-CSF expression is regulated by epidermal growth factor receptor, EGFR signaling, and transforming growth factor alpha (TGF-α); the first inhibits GM-CSF production, whereas the second upregulated this process.

TSLP plays an important role in AD, as it activates dendritic cells (DC) to produce chemokines such as thymus- and activation-regulated chemokine (TARC)/chemokine (C-C motif) ligand (CCL)17 and macrophage-derived chemokine/CCL22, leading to the infiltration of Th-2 cells infiltration in lesional AD skin (Pastore et al. 1997; Ong 2014).

3.3 Clinical Diagnosis of Atopic Eczema and Evaluation of Disease Severity

3.3.1 Clinical Diagnosis

The commonly used clinical diagnostic procedure in most western countries has been developed by Hanifin and Rajka (1980); it takes into account major and minor criteria, based on clinical experience. In the presence of a patient with a syndrome similar to that of AD, it is always important to think about the differential diagnosis. Scabies, which could be source of confusion when superimposed on a pre-existing AD, should be excluded. In addition, when considering skin inflammatory disorders in children, there are a number of conditions having similar clinical features with AD such as seborrheic dermatitis and other eczematous diseases that can be difficult to differentiate with AD (Champion et al. 1998).

3.3.2 Evaluation of Disease Severity of Atopic Dermatitis

As for other eczematous skin disorders (allergic contact dermatitis, contact urticaria, metal allergy, irritant contact dermatitis), there are a number of scoring systems used in practice to evaluate the severity of eczematous diseases. Below, a list of different eczema severity scoring systems is provided; however, only one of them (SCORAD) which is most commonly used is described.

1. SCORAD: SCORing Atopic Dermatitis (Fig. 3.2)

It is the most utilized clinical tool for the assessment of the extent and the severity of eczema before and after treatment. It is used by dermatologists and also specialists in the field of immunology and allergy, as well as occupational skin diseases. Two factors are taken into account during the assessment: area of affected body part and the intensity of skin lesions.

(a) **Area**: in order to determine the extent of the disease, the sites affected by eczema are shaded on a drawing of the body; the rule of 9 is used to calculate the affected area (A) as a percentage of whole body, as follows:

- Head and neck: 9%
- Upper limbs: 9% each
- Lower limbs: 18% each
- Anterior trunk: 18%
- Back: 18%
- Genitals: 1%

To have the total affected area (A), the scores of all affected areas should be added up. Note that a possible maximum for A is 100%.

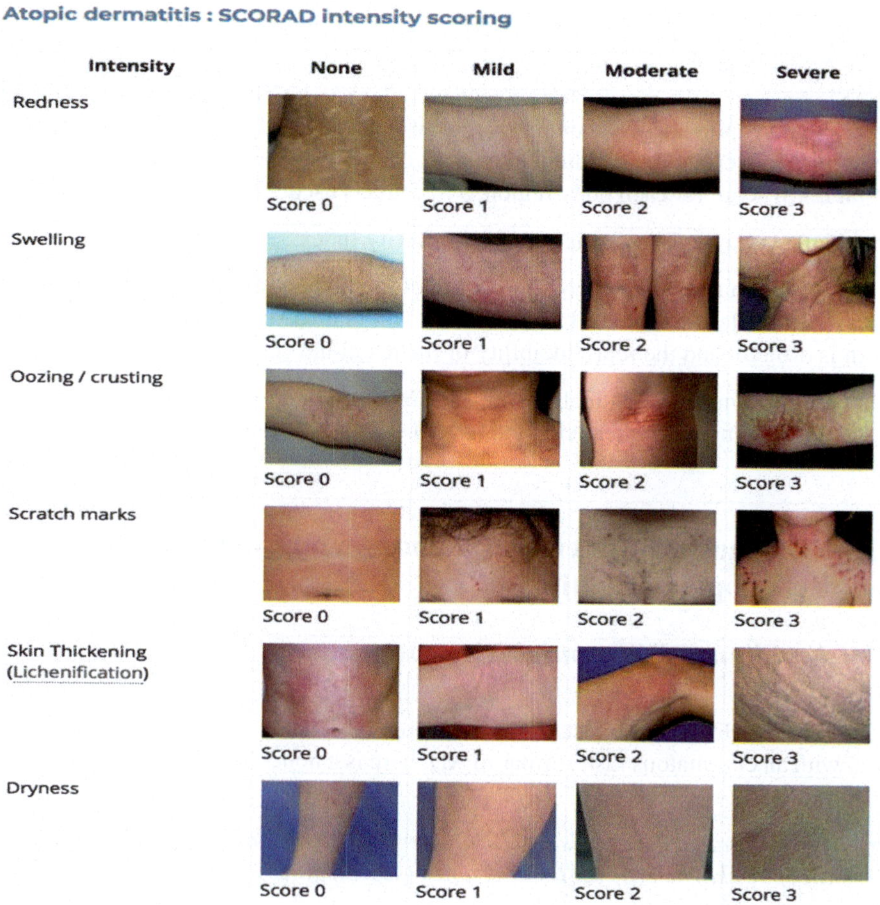

Fig. 3.2 Illustration of SCORAD system according to the intensity of objective skin signs (Oakley 2009). [©DermNet-New Zealand: https://creativecommons.org/licenses/by-nc-nd/3.0/nz/legalcode (original image not modified)]

(b) **Intensity**: first, a representative area is selected, and the intensity of each of these **six objective signs** "redness," "swelling," "oozing/crusting," "scratch marks," and "skin thickening or lichenification" is assessed in the selected body area as none (0), mild (1), moderate (2), or severe (3). The intensity scores are added together to give "*B*" (maximum = 18).

Then, the patient or his/her relative should assess the intensity of symptoms such as itch or pruritus and sleeplessness with the use of a visual analogue scale where 0 means "absence of itch" or no sleeplessness and 10 represents the worst imaginable itch or sleeplessness. These scores related to subjective symptoms are added to give "*C*" (20 being the maximum score). In order to determine the total AD severity or SCORAD score for an individual, here is the formula: **total score =** $A/5 + 7B/2 + C$ (Oakley 2009).

2. EASI: Eczema Area and Severity Index

EASI system is quite similar to SCORAD; in contrast to the SCORAD index, the EASI consists of the assessment of eczema extent on a scale of 0–6 in four defined body regions plus the assessment of the intensity of erythema, infiltration, and/or papulation, excoriation, and lichenification, each on a scale of 0–3. To calculate the total EASI score for each body region, a formula is used. The scores are then added.

3. ADASI: Atopic Dermatitis Area and Severity Index

The system uses a color-coding system of the body charts and point counting to produce a scale. A number of trials have shown that AD assessment using this system is difficult and the reproducibility of the result not certain.

4. Other scoring systems include the ADAM, the SIS, the ADSI, the SSS, and the SASSAD index (Eichenfield et al. 2017).

3.4 Diagnosis, Differential Diagnosis, and Complications of Atopic Dermatitis

3.4.1 Clinical Differential Diagnosis

Considering clinical manifestations, there are several other skin disorders that present with an eczematous rash similar to AD; here is a nonexhaustive list of those skin conditions:

- *Allergic contact dermatitis (ACD) and irritant contact dermatitis (ICD)*
- *Sarcoptic skin disease (SSD) or scabies* (see Chap. 13)
- *Seborrheic dermatitis*
- *Cutaneous T cell lymphoma*
- *Infantile psoriasis*
- *Primary immunodeficiency diseases*
- *Acrodermatitis enteropathica*
- *Nutritional deficiency (biotin, zinc)*
- *Ichthyosis vulgaris*
- *Drug reactions*

The clinician should have the necessary knowledge on the abovementioned skin disorders, remember the clinical diagnostic criteria (see Table 3.1), and be able to carefully conduct the evaluation of the localization and morphological characteristics of the skin rash, combined with patient's history, in order to make a sound diagnosis of the patient's condition (Thomsen 2014, Lyons et al. 2015).

A number of factors in the work or the living environment can complicate AD. However, the major complication is caused by *microorganisms* such as bacteria, viruses, and fungi. The colonization of AD skin by *Staphylococcus aureus* often

Table 3.1 The UK refinement of Hanifin and Rajka's diagnostic criteria for atopic dermatitis (scabies excluded)

Criteria that qualify a case of atopic dermatitis according to UK's Hanifin and Rajka diagnostic approach
• Presence of itchy skin (report of episodes of scratching or rubbing), plus three or more of the following
• Onset below 2 years of age (not applicable to a child who is aged less than 4)
• History of skin crease involvement (cheeks in children under 10 years included)
• History of generally dry skin
• Personal history of other atopic disease such as asthma and/or allergic rhinitis (or history of any atopic disease in a first-degree relative in children under 4 years)
• Visible flexural dermatitis (or dermatitis of the cheeks/forehead and outer limbs in children under 4 years)

The UK refinement of Hanifin and Rajka's diagnostic criteria (Williams et al. 1994)

occurs (about 90% of AD patients), which may cause *impetigo*, characterized by oozing lesions. In addition, the density of *S. aureus* on AD skin correlates directly with AD severity (Bath-Hextall et al. 2010; Lyons et al. 2015). In addition, studies have shown the presence of specific IgE to staphylococcal enterotoxin in sera of AD patients and that this specific IgE is associated with AD severity in children (Lin et al. 2000). On the other hand, a number of viruses can also aggravate AD. For example, *herpes simplex virus* (HSV-1 or HSV-2) can spread on AD skin and cause *eczema herpeticum*, with the presence of widespread vesicles localized to the face, upper chest, and scalp. The patient will present with fever, malaise, and lymphadenopathy. Another infectious complication is caused by the dissemination of *Coxsackie virus*, causing the "eczema coxsackium" (Mathes et al. 2013). Thus, preventing and treating these complications should be part of AD management strategies.

3.4.2 Skin Prick Test (SPT)

Skin prick test (SPT) (Fig. 3.3) is an essential test procedure that helps to confirm sensitization in IgE-mediated allergic disorders in AD subjects as well as individuals with asthma, anaphylaxis, allergic rhinoconjunctivitis, urticaria, and food and drug allergy. SPK is a reliable method that provides evidence for sensitization and to confirm the diagnosis of suspected type allergy (Heinzerling et al. 2013). SPT is less invasive and inexpensive; however, in order to obtain reliable and reproducible result, it is advised that a professional such as a dermatologist perform the test (Ebruster 1959; Heinzerling et al. 2013). The test is indicated in case of suspicion of type 1 allergy and also when screening for a predisposition to develop atopic diseases (AD, asthma, allergic rhinitis) in both adults and children.

The principle for SPT for skin allergens is that its interpretation utilizes the presence and the degree of skin reactivity as a surrogate marker for sensitization. Allergens are introduced into the skin, inducing a cross-link of specific IgE bound

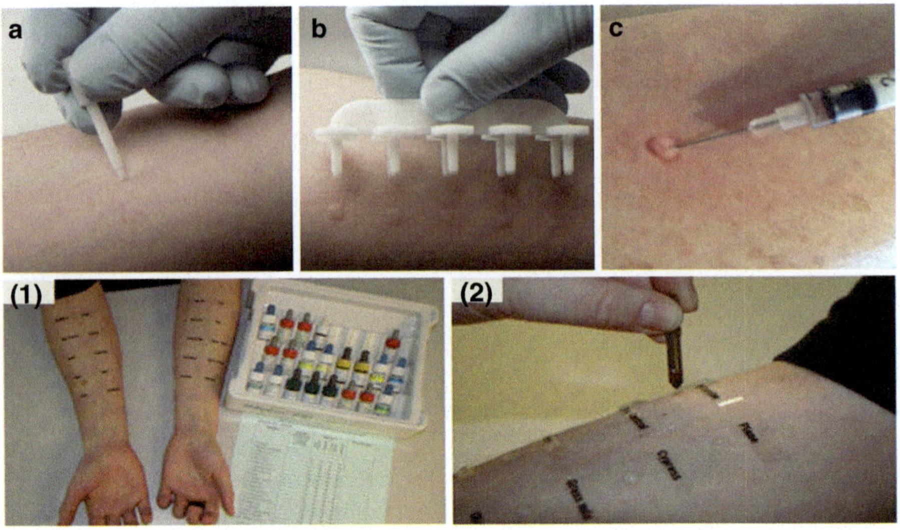

Fig. 3.3 Skin prick test procedures in two subjects performed by different specialists; **subject1**, examples of single-site (**a**) and multiple-site (**b**) skin prick testing and intradermal testing (**c**) (Fatteh et al. 2014) [©Fatteh et al.; licensee BioMed Central Ltd. 2014]; **subject2**, (1) preparation for skin prick test on the forearm. (2) Prick testing with lancet through a drop of allergen extract (Heinzerling et al. 2013) [© Heinzerling et al.; licensee BioMed Central Ltd. 2013]

to mast cell surface receptors, a consecutive mast cell degranulation, and the release of histamine and other mediators of allergic inflammation (Heinzerling et al. 2013). Although SPT is considered to be safe, there are precautions and contraindications that should be taken into account (checking expiration date of allergen extracts, use of proper positive and negative controls, chronic diseases such as renal failure or cancer which are among the factors that reduce skin test reactivity during SPT, difficulty to perform the test in patients with severe eczema, avoidance of SPT during pregnancy, in patients taking medication such as beta-blockers or angiotensin-converting enzyme (ACE) inhibitors, when tryptase levels are high which increase the risk of SPT-induced anaphylaxis, etc.) (Heinzerling et al. 2013).

3.5 Preventive Measures for Atopic Dermatitis

The rising AD incidence and its familial association have led to the search for prophylactic strategies. Obviously, AD cannot be prevented in all cases, but there is a possibility to attempt to reduce the risk of its development. In this section, preventive measures susceptible to possibly avoid AD development in predisposed individuals are presented, whereas conventional and alternative treatments are presented in Chap. 5 of this work. The most promising AD preventive agents are listed below:

1. Probiotics

Probiotics have been attracting the attention of many researchers in the field of allergy, given recent reports from clinical trials. A randomized controlled trial on 415 pregnant women who received probiotics (milk containing *Lactobacillus rhamnosus GG*, *Lactobacillus acidophilus La-5*, and *Bifidobacterium animalis* subsp. *lactis BB-12*) versus milk without probiotic from 36 weeks' gestation until 3 months postpartum showed a significant reduction in AD incidence among the offspring of probiotic-supplemented mothers (Sullivan and Silverberg 2017).

2. Emollients

   Another group of AD preventive agents that are being studied are emollients. Dry skin has been recognized as one of factors that impair skin barrier function and precede the onset of AD. Thus, the use of agents that prevent dry skin and enhance the skin barrier function is believed to be another way to reduce the risk of AD development in high-risk and even low-risk individuals (Uehara and Miyauchi 1984; Williams et al. 2012). A cohort study by Simpson et al. (2010) on emollients and primary prevention of AD showed promising results; only 15% (vs. 85%) of participants developed AD, and skin barrier measurements remained within normal ranges, suggesting a protective effect of emollient preparation used in this study as compared to historical controls. Furthermore, the same research team has conducted a randomized clinical trial to determine whether skin barrier enhancement from birth could prevent the onset of AD in neonates. It was found that emollient-treated neonates had a 50% reduction of AD development (Simpson et al. 2014).

3.6 Current Conventional Therapies for Atopic Dermatitis

Nowadays, considering the progress made in regard to research on AD, the management of this skin disorder is mainly based on targeting defects related to AD development, namely, the dysfunction of the skin barrier and the subsequent inflammation, along with the treatment of associated complications such as infections. The goal is to improve patient's quality of life (QOL) and prevent the occurrence of complications, which include drug-induced adverse effects (Lyons et al. 2015). In the following lines, we provide a list of commonly used therapies against AD and their anti-inflammatory mechanisms (other agents used as alternatives to corticosteroids and calcineurin inhibitors are discussed in another chapter of this book):

1. *Topical Corticosteroids*

   – They are considered as the most effective AD treatment. They are efficacious to treat acute flares related to AD and severe cases and also to reduce pruritus and maintain the control of the inflammation. Given the existence of different categories of corticosteroids that are in use, healthcare providers should consider to choose the drug based on the severity of the flares and the affected body area to make the care plan. For example, low-potency corticosteroids may be preferred to highly potent ones in case of mild AD, and one thing to always remember is that "the greater the potency, the higher the risk of local and systemic side effects!" For body areas with thinner skin, a lower-potency corticosteroid should be used, because in this case, there is a greater chance of absorption and higher risk of side effects, whereas for other body areas with normal skin thickness, a short course of higher-potency corticosteroid would achieve the control of AD flares.

- There is a wide range of potencies for corticosteroids; group 1 comprises the lowest potent drugs (e.g., *dexamethasone*, *hydrocortisone* 1% ointment), whereas group 7 has the most potent ones (e.g., topical *clobetasol propionate*, *fluticasone*, *mometasone*) (Lyons et al. 2015). Paller and Mancini (2011) provide a wide range and categories of currently used topical corticosteroids according to their relative potency.
- In children, it is advised to use the lowest-potency topical steroids in order to minimize the risk of side effects, whereas the use of corticosteroids on the face of any AD patient should be avoided. On the other hand, to treat moderate to severe AD (see SCORAD system), stepwise adjustment instructions regarding corticosteroid potency should be used while considering the severity of the flares and body areas involved.
- Although systemic corticosteroids may provide a rapid relief of AD flares, some researchers advise to avoid them for AD treatment, as their discontinuation often results in more severe AD (Lyons et al. 2015).
- Side effects include skin atrophy, adrenal insufficiency, acne, striae, telangiectasias, and infections.

2. *Topical Calcineurin Inhibitors*

- Their anti-inflammatory effect results from the selective blocking of cytokine transcription in activated T cells. These drugs serve as alternatives to topical corticosteroids. They work by inhibiting *calcineurin* in the skin, which regulates the activity of several transcription factors that control cell division and trigger the early stages of T cell activation. A number of randomized trials showed that treatment with those calcineurin inhibitors may take several weeks or months to improve atopic dermatitis patients' condition, and their use is not without adverse effects. Their major side effect is a transient burning that often occurs a few days after the start of treatment (Lebwohl and Gower 2006). These are often used when treating AD patients who require a long-term anti-inflammatory treatment.
- Two drugs from this group are currently in use in many countries: *pimecrolimus* (Elidel) and *tacrolimus* (Protopic).

3. *Antimicrobials*

- Given that the colonization of AD by *Staphylococcus aureus* often occurs, the treatment of this complication (infection) is included in some AD treatment guidelines, particularly for pediatric AD patients, for example, use of bleach baths.

4. *Systemic Treatment*
   - Systemic medications are becoming a prevalent therapeutic option for chronic and severe AD, and drugs considered as most efficacious are cyclosporine, methotrexate mofetil (MMF), and azathioprine (AZA) (Sidbury et al. 2014).
5. *Antihistamines*
   - Most AD patients complain of pruritus, the most common feature of this skin disorder, which is detrimental for their quality of life. In AD, pruritus results from a number of mediators such as neuropeptides and cytokines (e.g., IL-31), the reason why antihistamines may be ineffective to control pruritus; thus, some researchers have suggested that treatment should be focused on addressing barrier dysfunction and skin inflammation (Lyons et al. 2015).

3.7 Conclusion

AD prevalence is on the rise worldwide mainly due to changes in the living environment, given the role played by environmental factors in industrialized countries where high rates of AD have been reported. The discovery of filaggrin skin barrier gene and its role in the development of the disease have recently brought a focus on the gene-environment interactions, leading to the search for environmental triggers of AD in order to effectively ameliorate AD management. Therefore, in light of the foregoing, there is a crucial need to identify alternative adjuvant and therapeutic agents that could help to effectively prevent the development of AD in predisposed individuals and efficiently control disease symptoms in AD patients.

References

Alexander DD, Cabana MD. Partially hydrolyzed 100% whey protein infant formula and reduced risk of atopic dermatitis: a meta-analysis. J Pediatr Gastroenterol Nutr. 2010;50:422–30.

Bath-Hextall FJ, Birnie AJ, Ravenscroft JC, et al. Interventions to reduce Staphylo-coccus aureus in the management of atopic eczema: an updated Cochrane review. Br J Dermatol. 2010;163(1):12–26.

Benn CS, Melbye M, Wohlfahrt J, et al. Cohort study of sibling effect, infectious diseases, and risk of atopic dermatitis during first 18 months of life. BMJ. 2004;328:1223.

Blumenthal MN, Amos DM. Genetic and immunologic basis of atopic response. In: Champion RH, Burton JL, Burns DA, Breathnach SM, editors. Textbook of dermatology. London: Blackwell Science; 1998. p. 683–99.

Brown SJ, McLean WH. One remarkable molecule: Filaggrin. J Invest Dermatol. 2012;132(3 Pt 2):751–62.

Champion RH, Burton JL, Burns DA, Breathnach SM. Textbook of dermatology. 6th ed. London: Blackwell Science; 1998.
Coleman R, Trembath RC, Harper JI. Chromosome 11q13 and atopic eczema. Lancet. 1993;341(8853):1121–2.
Czamowicki T, Esaki H, Gonzales J, et al. Early pediatric atopic dermatitis shows only a cutaneous lymphocyte antigen (CLA)(+)TH2/TH1 cell imbalance, whereas adults acquire CLA(+) TH22/TC22 cell subsets. J Allergy Clin Immunol. 2015;136:941–51.
Darsow U, Lubbe J, Taieb A, et al. Position paper on the diagnosis and treatment of atopic dermatitis. J Eur Acad Dermatol Venereol. 2005;19:286–95.
De Benetto A, Rafaels NM, McGirt LY, et al. Tight junction defects in patients with atopic dermatitis. J Allergy Clin Immunol. 2011;127:773–86.e1-7.
Diepgen TL, Blettner M. Analysis of familial aggregation of atopic eczema and other atopic diseases by odds ratio regression models. In: Champion RH, Burton JL, Burns DA, Breathnach SM, editors. Textbook of dermatology. London: Blackwell Science; 1998. p. 683–99.
Doull IJ, Lawrence S, Watson M, et al. Allelic association of gene markers on chromosomes 5q and 11q with atopy and bronchial hyperresponsiveness. Am J Respir Crit Care Med. 1996;153(4):1280.
Ebruster H. The skin prick test, a recent cutaneous test for the diagnosis of allergic disorders. Wien Klin Wochenschr. 1959;71:551–4.
Eichenfield LF, Ahluwalia J, Waldman A, et al. Current guidelines for the evaluation and management of atopic dermatitis: a comparison of the Joint Task Force Practice Parameter and American Academy of Dermatology guidelines. J Allergy Clin Immunol. 2017;139(4S):S49–57.
Elias PM, Steinhoff M. "Outside-to-inside" (and back to "outside") pathogenic mechanisms in atopic dermatitis. J Invest Dermatol. 2008;128(5):1067–70.
Esaki H, Takeuchi S, Furusyo N, et al. Levels of immunoglobulin E specific to the major food allergen and chemokine (C-C motif) ligand (CCL)17/thymus and activation regulated chemokine and CCL22/macrophage-derived chemokine in infantile atopic dermatitis on Ishigaki Island. J Dermatol. 2016;43:1278–82.
Fatteh S, Rekkerth DJ, Hadley JA. Skin prick/puncture testing in North America: a call for standards and consistency. Allergy Asthma Clin Immunol. 2014;10:44.
Furue M, Kadono T. New therapies for controlling atopic itch. J Dermatol. 2015;42(9):847–50.
Furue M, Chiba T, Tsuji G, et al. Atopic dermatitis: immune deviation, barrier dysfunction, IgE autoreactivity and new therapies. Allergol Int. 2017;66:398–403.
Gittler JK, Shemer A, Suarez-Farinas M, et al. Progressive activation of T(h)2/T(h)22 cytokines and selective epidermal proteins characterizes acute and chronic atopic dermatitis. J Allergy Clin Immunol. 2012;130:1344–54.
Hanifin JM, Rajka RG. Diagnostic features of atopic dermatitis. Acta Derm Venereol (Stockh). 1980;92(144):44–7.
Heinzerling L, Mari A, Bergmann KC, et al. The skin prick test-European standards. Clin Transl Allergy. 2013;3:3.
Hidaka T, Ogawa E, Kobayashi EH, et al. The aryl hydrocarbon receptor AhR links atopic dermatitis and air pollution via induction of the neurotrophic factor artemin. Nat Immunol. 2017;18:64–73.
Irvine AD, McLean WH, Leung DY. Filaggrin mutations associated with skin and allergic diseases. N Engl J Med. 2011;365:1315–27.
Kawakami Y, Yumoto K, Kawakami T. An improved mouse model of atopic dermatitis and suppression of skin lesions by an inhibitor of Tec family kinases. Allergol Int. 2007;56:403–9.
Kim K. Influences of environmental chemicals on atopic dermatitis. Toxicol Res. 2015;31(2):89–96.
Kim J, Kim EH, Oh I, et al. Symptoms of atopic dermatitis are influenced by outdoor air pollution. J Allergy Clin Immunol. 2013;132(2):495–8.e1.
Kwan S, Burrows NP. Atopic dermatitis. Medicine. 2009;37(5):242–5.
Lebwohl M, Gower T. A safety assessment of topical calcineurin inhibitors in the treatment of atopic dermatitis. MedGenMed. 2006;8(4):8.

Lee HS, Kim SK, Han JB, et al. Inhibitory effects of Rumex japonicus Houtt. on the development of atopic dermatitis-like skin lesions in NC/Nga mice. Br J Dermatol. 2006;155:33–8.

Leung DY. Atopic dermatitis; new insights and opportunities for therapeutic intervention. J Allergy Clin Immunol. 2000;105:860–76.

Lin YT, Shau WY, Wang LF, et al. Comparison of serum specific IgE antibodies to staphylococcal enterotoxins between atopic children with and without atopic dermatitis. Allergy. 2000;55(7):641–6.

Lyons JJ, Milner JD, Stone KD. Atopic dermatitis in children: clinical features, pathophysiology and treatment. Immunol Allergy Clin North Am. 2015;35(1):161–83.

Marenholz I, Rivera VA, Esparza-Godillo J, et al. Association screening in the Epidermal Differentiation Complex (EDC) identifies an SPRR3 repeat number variant as a risk factor for eczema. J Invest Dermatol. 2011;131:1644–9.

Mascia F, Cataisson C, Lee TC, et al. EGFR regulates the expression of keratinocyte-derived granulocyte/macrophage colony-stimulating factor in vitro and in vivo. J Invest Dermatol. 2010;130(3):682–93.

Mathes EF, Oza V, Frieden IJ, et al. "Eczema coxsackium" and unusual cutaneous findings in an enterovirus outbreak. Pediatrics. 2013;132(1):e149–57.

Montnemery P, Nihlén U, Göran Löfdahl C, et al. Prevalence of self-reported eczema in relation to living environment, socio-economic status and respiratory symptoms assessed in a questionnaire study. BMC Dermatol. 2003;3:4.

Morar N, Cookson WO, Harper JI, et al. Filaggrin mutations in children with severe atopic dermatitis. J Invest Dermatol. 2007;127:1667–72.

Newell L, Polak ME, Perera J, et al. Sensitization via healthy skin programs Th2 responses in individuals with atopic dermatitis. J Invest Dermatol. 2013;133:2372.

Ngatu NR, Hirota R, Okajima MK, et al. Sacran, a natural skin barrier enhancer, improves atopic and contact eczema: Case report. Ann Phytomed. 2015;4(1):111–3.

Nickel RG, Casolaro V, Wahn U, et al. Atopic dermatitis is associated with a functional mutation in the promoter of the C-C chemokine RANTES. J Immunol. 2000;164:1612–6.

Nograles KE, Zaba LC, Shemer A, et al. Il-22-producing "T22" T cells account for upregulated IL-22 in atopic dermatitis despite reduced IL-17-producing TH17 T cells. J Allergy Clin Immunol. 2009;123:1244–52.

Nutten S. Atopic dermatitis: global epidemiology and risk factors. Ann Nutr Metab. 2015;66(1):8–16.

Nyembue TD, Vinck AS, Corvers K, et al. Sensitization to common aeroallergens in patients at an outpatient ENT clinic. B-ENT. 2011;7(2):79–85.

Oakley A. SCORAD (report 2009). 2009. Available from: https://www.dermnetnz.org/topics/scorad/ (Accessed 22 Nov 2017).

Oiso N, Fukai K, Ishii M. Interleukin 4 receptor alpha chain polymorphism Gln551Arg is associated with adult atopic dermatitis in Japan. Br J Dermatol. 2000;142:1003–6.

Ong PY. New insights in the pathogenesis of atopic dermatitis. Pediatr Res. 2014;75:171–5.

Paller AS, Mancini AJ. Chapter 3: Eczematous eruptions in childhood. In: Paller AS, Mancini AJ, editors. Hurwitz clinical pediatric dermatology. St Louis, MO: Elsevier Inc; 2011. p. 49.

Pastore S, Fanales-Belasio E, Albanesi C, et al. Granulocyte macrophage colony-stimulating factor is overproduced by keratinocytes in atopic dermatitis. Implications for sustained dendritic cell activation in the skin. J Clin Invest. 1997;99(12):3009–17.

Pénard-Morand C, Raherison C, Charpin D, et al. Long-term exposure to close-proximity air pollution and asthma and allergies in urban children. Eur Respir J. 2010;36(1):33–40.

Ruiz RG, Kemeny DM, Price JF. Higher risk of infantile atopic dermatitis from maternal atopy than from paternal atopy. Clin Exp Allergy. 1992;22:762–6.

Sandford AJ, Shirakawa T, Moffatt MF, et al. Localization of atopy and beta subunit of high-affinity IgE receptor (Fc epsilon RI) on chromosome 11q. Lancet. 1993;341:332–4.

Schafer T, Vieluf D, Behrendt H, et al. Atopic eczema and other manifestations of atopy: results of a study in East and West Germany. Allergy. 1996;51:532–9.

Seguchi T, Cui CY. Kusuda et al. Decreased expression of filaggrin in atopic skin. Arch Dermatol Res. 1996;288:442–6.
Sehgal VN, Khurana A, Mendiratta V, Saxena D, Srivastava G, Aggarwal AK. Atopic dermatitis; etio-pathogenesis, an overview. Indian J Dermatol. 2015;60(4):327–31.
Sidbury R, Davis DM, Cohen DE, et al. Guidelines of care for the management of atopic dermatitis: section 3. Management and treatment with phototherapy and systemic agents. J Am Acad Dermatol. 2014;71(2):327–49.
Simpson EL, Berry TM, Brown PA, et al. A pilot study of emollient therapy for primary prevention of atopic dermatitis. J Am Acad Dermatol. 2010;63(4):587.
Simpson EL, Chalmers JR, Hanifin JM, et al. Emollient enhancement of the skin barrier from birth offers effective dermatitis prevention. J Allergy Clin Immunol. 2014;134(4):818–23.
Song S, Lee K, Lee YM, et al. Acute health effects of urban fine and ultrafine particles on children with atopic dermatitis. Environ Res. 2011;111(3):394–9.
Strachan DP. Family size, infection and atopy: the first decade of the "hygiene hypothesis". Thorax. 2000;55:S2–S10.
Sugaya M, Morimura S, Suga H, et al. CCR4 is expressed on infiltrating cells in lesional skin of early mycosis fungoides and atopic dermatitis. J Dermatol. 2015;42:613–5.
Sullivan M, Silverberg NB. Current and emerging concepts in atopic dermatitis pathogenesis. Clin Dermatol. 2017;35(4):349–53.
Szajewska H, Horvath A. Meta-analysis of the evidence for a partially hydrolyzed 100% whey formula for the prevention of allergic diseases. Curr Med Res Opin. 2010;26:423–37.
Tesmer LA, Lundy SK, Sarkar S, Fox DA. Th17 cells in human disease. Immunol Rev. 2008;223:87–113.
Thomsen SF. Atopic dermatitis: natural history, diagnosis, and treatment. ISRN Allergy. 2014;2014:354250.
Uehara M, Miyauchi H. The morphologic characteristics of dry skin in atopic dermatitis. Arch Dermatol. 1984;120:186–90.
Williams H. Atopic dermatitis. N Engl J Med. 2005;352:2314–24.
Williams HC, Burney PGJ, Pembroke AC, et al. Working party's diagnostic criteria for atopic dermatitis III Independent hospital validation. Br J Dermatol. 1994;131:406–16.
Williams H, Robertson C, Stewart A, et al. Worldwide variations in the prevalence of symptoms of atopic eczema in the International Study of Asthma and Allergies in Childhood. J Allergy Clin Immunol. 1999;103(1 Pt 1):125–38.
Williams HC, Chalmers JR, Simpson EL. Prevention of atopic dermatitis. F1000 Med Rep. 2012;4:24.
Yemaneberhan H, Flohr C, Lewis SA, et al. Prevalence and associated factors of atopic dermatitis symptoms in rural and urban Ethiopia. Clin Exp Allergy. 2004;34:779–85.

Chapter 4
Occupational Contact Dermatitis

Nlandu Roger Ngatu

Abstract Occupational contact dermatitis (OCD) is a skin disorder characterized by a red, sore, or inflamed skin after a direct contact with a substance. It is either of allergic (ACD) or irritative (ICD) nature, and they account for over 90% of all work-related skin disorders. The most frequent causes of occupational ACD are metals (nickel, chrome, cobalt), resins (epoxy resin, acrylic resin), rubber-based materials, agrichemicals, and plants; it is mostly characterized by scaly red (erythema) to pink areas of elevated skin that can be papules and/or plaques, vesicles (or blisters), and pruritus (itch). ICD, the most common occupational skin disorder (OSD), is five times more frequent than ACD and is characterized by scaling, erythema, and a mild edema at the site of contact with the irritant substance. The differential diagnosis between ACD and ICD is made mainly based on the clinical features and, eventually, patch testing (when positive, ACD will be the diagnosis). If pruritus appears as the dominant symptom in ACD, however, ICD patients often have burning feeling and pain. Another clinical feature that may facilitate the diagnosis consists of the status of the border of the skin lesions (erythema). In case of ICD, borders are less distinct, whereas distinct lines, angles, and borders are characteristics of ACD. In occupational settings with risk of OCD, a number of preventives measures can be implemented to reduce the risk; they include *pre-employment screening* which can help to identify predisposed subjects, the use of *personal protective devices and creams* (appropriate gloves, mask, barrier cream, after-work cream, etc.), and *technical measures* and *work organization* in order to reduce exposure to the sensitizer or irritant substance. Regarding OCD treatment, therapy based on corticosteroids is the first choice. Ultraviolet B (UVB) therapy based on UVB (medium wave length) and psoralen plus UVA (PUVA) is reported to be beneficial particularly for hand dermatitis, whereas a systemic treatment can be recommended for very severe and recalcitrant OCD.

Keywords Allergic contact dermatitis · Contact dermatitis · Irritant contact dermatitis · Scoring of atopic dermatitis

---

N. R. Ngatu, M.D., Ph.D. (✉)
Graduate School of Medicine, International University of Health and Welfare (IUHW), Chiba, Japan

Graduate School of Public Health, International University of Health and Welfare (IUHW), Tokyo, Japan

N. R. Ngatu, M. Ikeda (eds.), *Occupational and Environmental Skin Disorders*,
https://doi.org/10.1007/978-981-10-8758-5_4

List of Abbreviations

ACD	Allergic contact dermatitis
ICD	Irritant contact dermatitis
OCD	Occupational contact dermatitis
OSH	Occupational safety and health
PUVA	Psoralen plus ultraviolet A
UVB	Ultraviolet

4.1 Introduction

4.1.1 Definition of Occupational Contact Dermatitis

Occupational contact dermatitis (OCD) or occupational contact eczema is an inflammatory skin condition characterized by a red, sore, or inflamed skin after a direct contact with a substance. The disease can also be caused by a factor in the living environment. OCD impact the workers' quality of life and workability. It is a common skin disease in industrial countries with a considerable socioeconomic impact (Coenraads and Goncalo 2007).

4.1.2 Epidemiology of Occupational Contact Dermatitis

It has been reported that OCD accounts for 90% of all cases of work-related skin disorders (Sasseville 2008; Clark and Zirwas 2009). There are two categories of this skin disorder, occupational allergic (ACD) and occupational irritant contact dermatitis (ICD). In the United States, it has been reported that high rates of OCD are observed in occupational settings such as mining, natural resources, manufacturing, and health services (US Department of Labor 2010; Usatine and Riojas 2010). In 2004, occupational ICD accounted for 95% of all reported occupational skin diseases in the United States, whereas, in the same year, contact dermatitis accounted for 9.2 million hospital visits (Taylor and Amado 2010).

Additionally, an interview survey conducted to determine a 12-month OCD prevalence among 30,074 American workers showed a rate of 1700 per 100,000 (Behrens et al. 1994). In Europe, OCD prevalence rate of 6–10% has been reported, with a wide variation according to occupations (Belsito 2005, Bordel-Gomez et al. 2010, Codruta-Dana and Alexandru 2015). In China, a recent study conducted among 529 employees of a clothing manufacturing factory showed an overall OCD prevalence rate of 28.5%, with ironing workers being the most affected, 50.0%, followed by sewers (31.7%) (Chen et al. 2017).

It is important to note that the allergic and irritant nature of the contact dermatitis are difficult to distinguish by clinical and histological features. Moreover, the dermatitis-causing substance may also have both irritant and sensitizing effects on the skin. Furthermore, it is noteworthy that an irritant substance also harms the skin barrier function, which ipso facto promotes sensitization by enabling an increase of allergen absorption (Berard et al. 2003; Geraut et al. 2011).

4.2 Occupational Allergic Contact Dermatitis

4.2.1 Definition and Clinical Manifestations

Occupational allergic contact dermatitis or occupational ACD is a skin condition defined as a delayed hypersensitivity reaction, occurring 48–72 h after exposure to an allergen. In case of ACD, the skin changes occur after a reexposure to the same foreign substance (Usatine and Riojas 2010). The disease is responsible for 20% of cases of occupational dermatitis and may occur on any location of the body surface; the most frequent symptoms are scaly red (erythema) to pink areas of elevated skin that can be papules and/or plaques, vesicles (or blisters), and pruritus (itch) (Sasseville 2008).

4.2.2 Causes, Risk Factors, and Occupations at Risk

Humans can develop occupational ACD after a contact with a substance within the work environment, such as exposure to products containing nickel, chrome, and cobalt among miners, metal processing factory workers, jewelry workers, and dental hygienists (Table 4.1). Worldwide, nickel sulfate is reported to be the main cause of occupational ACD, particularly in women. Exposure to nickel, chromate, and cobalt is known as one of the main causes of occupational contact allergy (Thyssen 2011; Qin and Lampe 2015). A study on patch test reactivity among 14, 464 Italian patients with suspected ACD showed a high rate of nickel sulfate sensitization (24.6%), followed by cobalt chloride (10.2%) and potassium dichromate (8.7%). In addition, positive associations were found between nickel exposure and metal/mechanical work, between chromate and building trade work, and also between cobalt exposure and textile-, leather-, and cleaning-related occupations (Rui et al. 2010) (Table 4.1).

Another study conducted in Spain has shown a relatively high involvement of nickel sulfate (25.8%), followed by chromates (5.3%), cobalt chloride (5.1%), fragrance blends (4.6%), and balsam of Peru (4.4%) (Sasseville 2008; Garcia-Gavin et al. 2011). On the other hand, a prospective study carried out in Dakar, Senegal, showed a prevalence of occupational ACD of 12.9%, involving exposure in occupational settings such as construction sites, mechanics, healthcare settings, cleaning and trade services; and the main causal agents were chromates (construction work), *N*-isopropyl *N*-phenyl-paraphenylenediamine, fragrance mix, thiuram mix, colophane, formaldehyde and nickel sulfate (Niang et al. 2007).

Table 4.1 Highly frequent occupational causes of allergic contact dermatitis (ACD) (Modified from Dobashi et al. 2017)

Agent/product	Clinical features and workers at risk
Metals (nickel, chrome, cobalt)	Those metals often cause ACD that may extend beyond the contact site. The disease occurs after a skin contact with product containing nickel, chrome, or cobalt (accessories, leather, coating materials, etc.). Miners, metal processing factory and industry workers, jewelry workers, dental hygienists, etc. are among workers at risk (Sasseville 2008; Rui et al. 2010; Thyssen 2011; Qin and Lampe 2015)
Resin, epoxy resin, acrylic resin	Epoxy and acrylic resins have numerous industrial applications as hardeners, plasticizers, and additives; they are widely used in household environment (e.g., plastic materials) and are well-known as a skin sensitizer responsible for ACD among painters, metal processing workers, construction workers, etc. (Tosti et al. 1993; Rademaker 2000; Qin and Lampe 2015)
Rubber (MBT, TMTD)	In some work settings (healthcare workers, laboratory workers, mechanics, etc.), rubber gloves and boots may cause allergic reaction characterized with erythema and lichenification (Qin and Lampe 2015)
Cutting oil, machine oil	Cutting oil and other types of oil used, for example, as lubricants contain chemicals that may cause ACD (Niklasson et al. 1993)
Agrichemicals (herbicides, antibacterial agents)	Chemicals used in farms to reduce wild herbs/grass or agents used to disinfect crops may cause skin sensitization. Farming and food processing are among occupations at risk (Qin and Lampe 2015)
Plant materials and compounds	There are a number of plant materials or compounds that induce contact allergy. For example, urushiol in Japanese wax tree, *Toxicodendron sylvestre, Toxicodendron trichocarpum*, poison ivy, and poison oak are incriminated in cases of ACD. *Ginkgolic acid* and *bilobol* from *Ginkgo biloba* tree and also *alantolactone*, *arteglasin A* from sunflower, *Artemisia*, lettuce, Margaret, and *Dahlia* can also cause skin allergy (Dobashi et al. 2017)

ACD allergic contact dermatitis, *MBT* mercaptobenzothiazole, *TMTD* tetramethyl thiuram disulfide (both MBT and TMTD are known as rubber accelerators). The table shows the most frequent causes of ACD in occupational settings; a longer list of environmental and occupational skin sensitizers is provided in Chap. 2 of this book

Besides, a number of chemical agents are also incriminated in the occurrence of ACD, such as resins, rubber, cutting and machine oil, agrichemicals, and plant-derived materials and compounds (Qin and Lampe 2015) (Table 4.1).

There are numerous endogenous and exogenous factors influencing the development of contact dermatitis (Taylor and Amado 2010):

(a) *Endogenous factors*:

- Atopic status, individual susceptibility, age, skin permeability, race, sensitivity of ultraviolet light, and lack of hardening

(b) *Exogenous factors*:

- Environment (temperature, humidity), body temperature, properties of the chemical agent (pH, chemical activity), mechanical factors (abrasion, friction, pressure, etc.), duration of the exposure, direct contact vs. airborne contact, and the use of protective device or garments

4.2.3 Clinical Manifestations of Allergic Contact Dermatitis

ACD can occur in a human at any age and in individuals of any ethnical or racial background. Individuals with a skin condition (such as stasis dermatitis, otitis externa, or pruritus ani) requiring frequent application of topical agents can develop ACD over time. Most ACD patients complain of itch and discomfort. However, some patients will visit the doctor based on the appearance of skin rash. In acute cases, ACD patients will have erythema, scaly red or pink areas of elevated skin (plaques or papules), vesicles, and bullae, whereas chronic cases may involve lichen, fissures, and cracks (Usatine and Riojas 2010). In case of ACD, individual skin lesions often have distinct borders and a geometric shape with straight edges and sharp angles.

4.3 Occupational Irritant Contact Dermatitis

4.3.1 Definition and Epidemiology

Irritant contact dermatitis (ICD) is an inflammation of the skin at the place of contact with a chemical substance. Occupational ICD is the most common occupational skin disorder (OSD); it is five times more frequent than ACD and represents approximately 50–80% of all OSD (Nosbaum et al. 2009). ICD consists of an inflammation of the skin that is generally manifested by scaling, erythema, and a mild edema. It is a nonspecific response of the skin to direct chemical damage which causes a release of inflammatory mediators mainly from epidermal cells. Among the causes, there are corrosive agents that cause the death of epidermal cells; skin ulcer or burn are its main clinical manifestations. Extreme pH, detergents, and organic solvents are among the main causes (Mathias and Maibach 1978; Broberg et al. 1990; Morris-Jones et al. 2002).

4.3.2 Etiology and Clinical Manifestations of Occupational Irritant Contact Dermatitis

Of the substances that causes ACD, some can also be responsible for ICD. Common irritant chemical agents that cause ICD include:

- Acids (sulfuric acid, nitric acid, hydrochloric acid, chromic acid, hydrofluoric acid)
- Alkalis (calcium, sodium, sodium cyanide, potassium cyanide, potassium hydroxide)
- Organic solvent

- Detergents

Besides the above factors, others may also cause ICD, such as:

- Wet work (it is considered the leading cause of ICD)
- Degreasing agents
- Dusts (mineral and organic dusts)
- Friction
- Animal products, Cosmetics
- Low humidity
- Topical medications
- Tear gas
- Metalworking fluids

In chronic cumulative ICD cases (with weak irritant chemicals), the patient will mostly present with itch, skin dryness, erythema, hyperkeratosis, and fissures, in addition, oozing, crusts, and cracks. However, in case of acute ICD (the second and major type of disease) resulting from exposure of the skin to strong irritant chemicals such as alkalis and acids, the patient often presents with the following skin lesions: erythema, vesicles, edema, vesicles, and tissue necrosis (English 2004; Taylor and Amado 2010).

4.4 Differential Diagnosis of Occupational Contact Dermatitis

4.4.1 Differential Diagnosis Based on Clinical Features

In order to make the differential diagnosis between contact dermatitis and endogenous eczema, and also between ACD and ICD, patient history and the determination of the causative substance are crucial not only for a good management of the disease but also to prevent further damages and implement control measures to reduce the risk. A number of clinical features can help to distinguish ACD from ICD, as shown in Table 4.2. ICD skin lesions can appear on any area of the body where the contact with the irritant substance occurred; but most of the times, the disease occurs on hands (hand eczema). On the other hand, ACD lesions often appear on the exposed

Table 4.2 Clinical features that distinguish occupational ICD from ACD

Clinical feature	Irritant	Allergic
Location	Hands mainly	Most often, exposed areas of skin
Symptoms	Burning, pruritus (itch), pain	Pruritus (itch) is a dominant symptom
Surface appearance	Dry and fissured skin	Vesicles and bullae
Lesion borders	Less distinct borders	Distinct angles, lines, and borders

ACD allergic contact dermatitis, *ICD* irritant contact dermatitis (Usatine and Riojas 2010)

body area. Additionally, if ACD is mainly characterized by pruritus as dominant symptom, patients often have burning feeling and pain. Another clinical feature that may facilitate the diagnosis consists of the status of border of the skin lesions (erythema or skin rash). In case of ICD, borders are less distinct, whereas distinct lines, angles, and borders are characteristics of ACD (Liccardi et al. 2002) (Table 4.2).

4.4.2 Patch Test

Patch test, which has high sensitivity and specificity (70–80%), represents the main diagnostic tool for the confirmation of ACD. The test is mostly performed by a dermatologist and consists of the application of antigen to the skin at standardized concentrations and in an appropriate vehicle and under occlusion. The body area that is most commonly used for patch testing is the back. In general, 2 days (48 h) later, the individual who underwent patch testing should be reexamined to see if any reaction to any of the tested substances occurred; again, a further 2 days later, the skin examination is performed to check whether the subject may have a delayed reaction to any of the substances.

Recent "S1-Guidelines of the German Contact Allergy Group (GKG)" (Brasch et al. 2014) provide some modifications and additions to patch testing as follows:

1. For "strip" patch test, they recommend a reduction of the horny layer prior to allergen application.
2. For the repeated open application test (ROAT), a suspected allergen is repeatedly applied openly over several days.
3. Additional scratch testing can be helpful when adequate transepidermal administration of the test substance is not possible when performing patch testing; also delayed readings of test results over several days can be envisaged.
4. Prick test (intracutaneous testing) can be helpful in case of suspicion of a protein contact allergy; here again, delayed readings are required.

4.5 Prevention and Treatment of Occupational Contact Dermatitis

New guidelines for OCD management from the Japanese Society of Allergology (JSA) emphasize the importance of the identification of the cause (allergen or irritant substance) following the onset of the disease. When the etiology is determined, a notification should be sent to the person in charge of workers' safety and health in the work setting or the employer so that necessary assessments and interventions be implemented in order to control the exposure and protect the health of other workers.

Table 4.3 Preventive measures for occupational contact dermatitis

General preventive measures for OCD
• *Pre-employment screening* (check personal history, atopic status, know allergens, etc.)
• *Personal protection*:
–Appropriate gloves, masks, or other protective device
–Barrier cream
–After-work cream
• *Technical measures* (change of work procedures to reduce risk, automation, etc.)
• *Work organization* (reduce exposure)

Table 4.3 is based on report from English JSC (2004) (details are provided in Chap. 2)

4.5.1 Prevention of Occupational Contact Dermatitis

Prior to employment, the employer should check whether a person applying for the job is fit for the task and whether products or substances used at work might cause nuisance to the applicant. That is because some individuals have predisposing factors for ACD or ICD. In a work setting, an inventory of health hazards should be performed and each worker should be informed on safety conditions at his/her workstation. In order to prevent the exposure to a sensitizer or irritant substance present in the work environment, its elimination should be envisaged. When that is not feasible for any reason, the use of appropriate protective tools or devices should be recommended (gloves, mask, protective garments, etc.). On the other hand, for workers with possible occupational exposure to chemical substances, topical application of barrier creams or after-work creams may confer protection against skin irritants. Moreover, changing work procedures in way that reduce duration of exposure, for example, and educating or training workers to increase awareness of potential skin hazards may help to reduce exposure to the hazard (Table 4.3).

4.5.2 Treatment of Occupational Contact Dermatitis

As for other inflammatory skin disorders, the administration of a therapeutic agent is tailored to the severity of the dermatitis, and hydrophilic preparations such as cream, lotion, or gel should be preferred in case of acute dermatitis, whereas chronic dermatitis will mostly require water-in-oil-based preparations (ointment). The new "German Contact Dermatitis Guideline" (Brasch et al. 2014) proposes the following agents:

1. *Corticosteroids*: they represent the first-choice medication for symptomatic treatment; class II and class III corticosteroids are efficacious and mostly preferred in case of acute ACD. More importantly, the selection of suitable drug is made on the basis of the location of skin lesions (affected body area), the severity

of the dermatitis. Also, one should bear in mind corticosteroid-associated adverse effects and take them into account when making decision upon the type and the duration of the treatment. Also, one should remember that, in case of ICD treatment, weaker corticosteroids may not be effective.

2. *Calcineurin inhibitors*: in some European countries, these drugs (e.g., *tacrolimus* and *pimecrolimus*) are approved only for AD treatment, whereas in the United States, they are quite widely used. In Japan, they are often prescribed in AD patients only in case of corticosteroid contraindications.
3. *Ultraviolet (UVB) therapy*: UVB (medium wave length) and psoralen plus UVA (PUVA) are reported to be effective particularly in the treatment of chronic hand dermatitis (Petering et al. 2004; Stege 2008; Brasch et al. 2014).
4. *Systemic treatment*: in case topical treatment reveals to be ineffective, a systemic treatment is approved in some countries, but not without caution. Side effects specific to each drug should be taken into account. Currently, cyclosporine is the drug recommended by the German S1 guidelines as the first choice for severe and recalcitrant AD and hand dermatitis (Brasch et al. 2014).

4.6 Conclusion

Occupational contact dermatitis remains the most prevalent work-related skin disorder worldwide, with higher incidence (5–19 cases/10,000) in full-time workers annually and high rates of absenteeism and huge economic impact (Sadagopan et al. 2017). Increasing workers' awareness in regard to skin health hazards, the early detection of hazardous substances at workplace, the early diagnosis of the disease in affected workers, and the use of the expertise of skilled healthcare professionals in the field of occupational safety and health (OSH) are indispensable for the prevention and the control of occupational ACD and ICD.

References

Behrens V, Seligman P, Cameron L, et al. The prevalence of back pain, hand discomfort, and dermatitis in the US working population. Am J Public Health. 1994;84(11):1780–5.

Belsito DV. Occupational contact dermatitis: etiology, prevalence, and resultant impairment/disability. J Am Acad Dermatol. 2005;532:303–13.

Berard F, Marty JP, Nicolas JF. Allergen penetration through the skin. Eur J Dermatol. 2003;13(4):324–30.

Bordel-Gomez MT, Miranda-Romero A, Castrodeza-Sanz J. Epidemiology of contact dermatitis: prevalence of sensitization to different allergens and associated factors. Actas Dermosifiliogr. 2010;1012:196.

Brasch J, Becker D, Aberer W, et al. Guideline contact dermatitis. S1-Guidelines of the German Contact Allergy Group (DKG) of the German Dermatology Society (DDG), the Information Network of Dermatological Clinics (IVDK), the German Society for Allergology and Clinical Immunology (DGAKI), the Working Group for Occupational and Environmental

Dermatology (ABD) of the DDG, the Medical Association of German Allergologists (AeDA), the Professional Association of German Dermatologists (BVDD) and the DDG. Allergo J Int. 2014;23(4):126–38.
Broberg A, Kalimo K, Lindbald B, et al. Parental education in the treatment of childhood atopic eczema. Acta Derm Venereol (Stockh). 1990;70:495–9.
Chen YX, Cheng HY, Li LF. Prevalence and risk factors of contact dermatitis among clothing manufacturing employees in Beijing: a cross-sectional study. Medicine. 2017;96(12):e6356.
Clark SC, Zirwas MJ. Management of occupational dermatitis. Dermatol Clin. 2009;27(3):365–83.
Codruta-Dana P, Alexandru T. Prevalence of contact dermatitis among occupational and work-related diseases. Correlation between atopy and allergic or irritative contact dermatitis. Acta Medica Marisiensis. 2015;61(4):320–3.
Coenraads PJ, Goncalo M. Skin diseases with high public health impact. Contact dermatitis. Eur J Dermatol. 2007;17(6):1128–34.
Dobashi K, Akiyama K, Usami A, et al. Japanese guidelines for occupational allergic diseases 2017. Allergol Int. 2017;66(2):265–80.
English JSC. Current concepts of irritant contact dermatitis. Occup Environ Med. 2004;61:722–6.
Garcia-Gavin J, Armario-Hita JC, Fernandez-Redondo V, et al. Epidemiology of contact dermatitis in Spain. Results of the Spanish surveillance system on contact allergies for the year 2008. Actas Dermosifiliogr. 2011;102(2):98–105.
Geraut C, Geraut L, Jover H, et al. Occupational diseases due to cooling fluids. Eur J Dermatol. 2011;21(2):162–9.
Liccardi G, Dente B, Triggiani M, et al. A multicenter evaluation of the CARLA system for the measurement of specific IgE antibodies vs. other different methods and skin prick tests. J Invest Allergol Clin Immunol. 2002;12(4):235–41.
Mathias CG, Maibach HI. Dermatotoxicology monographs I. Cutaneous irritation: factors influencing the response to irritants. Clin Toxicol. 1978;13(3):333–46.
Morris-Jones R, Robertson SJ, White IR, et al. Dermatitis caused by physical irritants. Br J Dermatol. 2002;147(2):270–5.
Niang SO, Cisse M, Gaye FM, et al. Occupational allergic contact dermatitis in Dakar. Mali Med. 2007;22(3):34–7.
Niklasson B, Bjorkner B, Sundberg K. Contact allergy to a fatty acid ester component of cutting fluids. Contact Dermatitis. 1993;28(5):265–7.
Nosbaum A, Vocanson M, Rozieres A, et al. Allergic and irritant contact dermatitis. Eur J Dermatol. 2009;19(4):325–32.
Petering H, Breuer C, Herbst R, et al. Comparison of localized high-dose UVA1 irradiation versus topical cream psoralen-UVA for treatment of chronic vesicular dyshidrotic eczema. J Am Acad Dermatol. 2004;50:68–72.
Qin R, Lampe HP. Review of occupational contact dermatitis-Top allergens, best avoidance measures. Curr Treat Options Allergy. 2015;2(4):349–64.
Rademaker M. Occupational epoxy resin allergic contact dermatitis. Australas J Dermatol. 2000;41(4):222–4.
Rui F, Bovenzi M, Prodi A, et al. Nickel, cobalt and chromate sensitization and occupation. Contact Dermatitis. 2010;62(4):225–31.
Sadagopan K, Kalappan D, Sivaprakasam N, et al. Patch test results from an occupational and contact dermatitis clinic in a tertiary care hospital of southern India: a retrospective study. J Clin Diagn Res. 2017;11(8):WC11–4.
Sasseville D. Occupational contact dermatitis. Allergy Asthma Clin Immunol. 2008;4(2):59–65.
Stege H. Ultraviolet therapy for hand chronic dermatitis (published in German). Hautarzt. 2008;59:696–702.
Taylor JS, Amado A. Contact dermatitis and related conditions. Center for Continuing Education Report. 2010. http://www.clevelandclinicmeded.com/medicalpubs/diseasemanagement/dermatology/contact-dermatitis-and-related-conditions/. Accessed 10 Dec 2017.

Thyssen JP. Nickel and cobalt allergy before and after nickel regulation-evaluation of a public health intervention. Contact Dermatitis. 2011;65:1): 1–68.
Tosti A, Guerra L, Vincenzi C, et al. Occupational skin hazards from synthetic plastics. Toxicol Ind Health. 1993;9(3):493–502.
US Department of Labor. Workplace injuries and illnesses in 2008. 2010. http://www.bls.gov.news.release/pdf/osh.pdf. Accessed 12 Dec 2017.
Usatine RP, Riojas M. Am Fam Physician. 2010;82(3):249–55.

Chapter 5
Quality of Work Environment and Frequency of Work-Related Dermatitis Among Dust-Exposed African Informal Coltan Miners

Ngombe Leon-Kabamba, Nlandu Roger Ngatu, Etongola Papy Mbelambela, Melaku Haile Likka, Sakatolo Jean-Baptiste Kakoma, Numbi Oscar Luboya, Roger Wumba, and Brigitta Danuser

Abstract Work-related dermatitis (WRD) represents a broad range of skin conditions such as irritant (ICD) and allergic contact dermatitis (ACD), as well as atopic eczema, that are either caused by or exacerbated by activities at work. In 2010,

---

N. Leon-Kabamba, M.D., MPH.
Department of Public Health, Faculty of Medicine, University of Kamina, Kamina, Congo

N. R. Ngatu, M.D., Ph.D. (✉)
Graduate School of Medicine, International University of Health and Welfare (IUHW), Chiba, Japan

Graduate School of Public Health, International University of Health and Welfare (IUHW), Tokyo, Japan

E. P. Mbelambela, M.D., M.Sc.
Department of Environmental Medicine, Kochi Medical School, Kochi University, Nankoku, Japan

M. H. Likka
Department of Healthcare Information Science, Kochi Medical School, Kochi University, Nankoku, Japan

S. J.-B. Kakoma, M.D., Ph.D.
School of Public Health, University of Lubumbashi, Lubumbashi, Congo

N. O. Luboya, M.D., Ph.D.
Department of Public Health, Faculty of Medicine, University of Kamina, Kamina, Congo

School of Public Health, University of Lubumbashi, Lubumbashi, Congo

R. Wumba, M.D., Ph.D.
Department of Tropical Medicine, Faculty of Medicine, University of Kinshasa, Kinshasa, Congo

B. Danuser, M.D., Ph.D.
Service of Occupational Medicine, Institute for Work and Health, University of Lausanne and Geneva, Epalinges-Lausanne, Switzerland

N. R. Ngatu, M. Ikeda (eds.), *Occupational and Environmental Skin Disorders*,
https://doi.org/10.1007/978-981-10-8758-5_5

WRD affected 15.2 million American workers, representing 9.8% of the US working population. In 2016, we conducted the first "Congo Coltan Miners' Health Study." The present report comprises findings related to WRD. Here, data from 398 workers (199 coltan miners matched to 199 unexposed office workers) are reported. Workstation air quality (PM2.5 and volatile organic compounds or VOC levels) was monitored using BRAMC Air Quality Monitor BR-AIR-329. Each participant answered two questionnaires related to skin and respiratory health. Higher PM2.5 levels were detected at coltan miners' workstations as compared with control sites (range, 180–210 μg/m^3 vs. 19–44 μg/m^3, respectively; $p < 0.001$); similarly, higher VOC levels were also found in coltan miners' workstations (range, 1.4–2.3 vs. 0.5–0.8, respectively; $p < 0.05$). Additionally, markedly higher proportion of miners reported dermatitis for the last 12-month period (37% vs. 7%) and in the previous years as compared with controls (36.2% vs. 7%, respectively; $p < 0.001$). Furthermore, coltan mining work was strongly associated with WRD in the last 12-month period (aOR = 4.88 ± 1.15; 95% CI, 2.06–11.33) and in the previous years (aOR = 9.48 ± 12.3; 95% CI, 3.74–120.49). This first study on African informal coltan miners' health showed striking results, with high dust exposure levels (PM2.5, VOC) and high frequency of WRD, suggesting the necessity to implement dust control measures to improve occupational safety in coltan mining settings.

Keywords Africa · Coltan miner · Particulate matter · Tantalum · Volatile organic compound · Work-related dermatitis

Abbreviations

ACD	Allergic contact dermatitis
ICD	Irritant contact dermatitis
PM	Particulate matter
PPE	Personal protective equipment
VOC	Volatile organic compound
WRD	Work-related dermatitis

5.1 Introduction

5.1.1 Work-Related Dermatitis in the Mining Sector

The term *work-related dermatitis* (WRD) includes a broad range of skin conditions such as irritant (ICD) and allergic contact dermatitis (ACD), as well as atopic eczema that are either caused by or exacerbated by activities at work. WRD affected 15.2 million American workers (9.8% of working population) in 2010, according to a national health interview survey (Luckhaupt et al. 2013; St. Louis et al. 2014). In the United States, the mining sector has one of the highest incidence rates of occupational skin disorders among all industries of which OCD is the most prevalent, accounting for 9.2 million hospital visits in 2004 (US Department of Labor 2010; Taylor and Amado 2010; Poplin et al. 2005).

Exposure to airborne dust can cause dermatitis (Belsito 2005); and mining is an occupation that has been recognized as being arduous liable to injury and disease since ancient times. Workers involved in open-pit and underground mining are exposed to numerous health hazards, mainly of physical (traumatic agents, noise, heat, humidity, vibration) and chemical (silica and other types of dusts) nature (Donoghue 2004). The Democratic Republic of Congo (DRC), a country of the central African region, is home to a vast mineral wealth, with huge untapped deposits of raw minerals such as coltan (tantalum), cobalt, copper, diamond, and tin; thus, DRC's economy is mineral dependent (Yager 2016). The country's eastern Kivu provinces (which represent the battleground for the long-standing and recurrent armed conflicts since 1997) and the southern province of Katanga are reported to have the greatest coltan reserves in the world. From coltan ore, tantalum and niobium are extracted, separated, and refined into metals. Tantalum is used as powder (50%) to make capacitors, whereas the rest (15%) serves in processing foil and wire for capacitors; all of them are incorporated in electronic equipment (computer, mobile phones, etc.) (Sutherland 2011).

5.1.2 Objectives of the Study

In general, informal coltan mining is carried out with bare hands and without any safety equipment to protect miners from dust (Kabamba et al. 2016). To our knowledge, there have been no scientific reports on occupational safety and health of coltan miners in the medical literature. We evaluated the effects of chronic dust exposure on coltan miners' health. Here, we report on the frequency and predictors of contact dermatitis in dust-exposed informal coltan miners from Haut-Lomami (formerly Katanga Province), DRC.

5.2 Materials and Methods

5.2.1 Study Site, Design, Participants, and Questionnaires

This was a cross-sectional analytical study conducted in Malemba-Nkulu District, Haut-Lomami (Fig. 5.1a) in DRC, a country located in the central Africa region (Fig. 5.1b), from August 1 through September 2016. In total, 441 Congolese workers (including 199 coltan miners and 242 office workers) who have been working for at least a year and accepted to sign the informed consent form were enrolled in the study. For controls (office workers), those who had any other activity with dust exposure were excluded. The final study sample for the present report comprises 199 coltan miners and 199 controls ($N = 398$) matched by age and the category of body mass index (BMI).

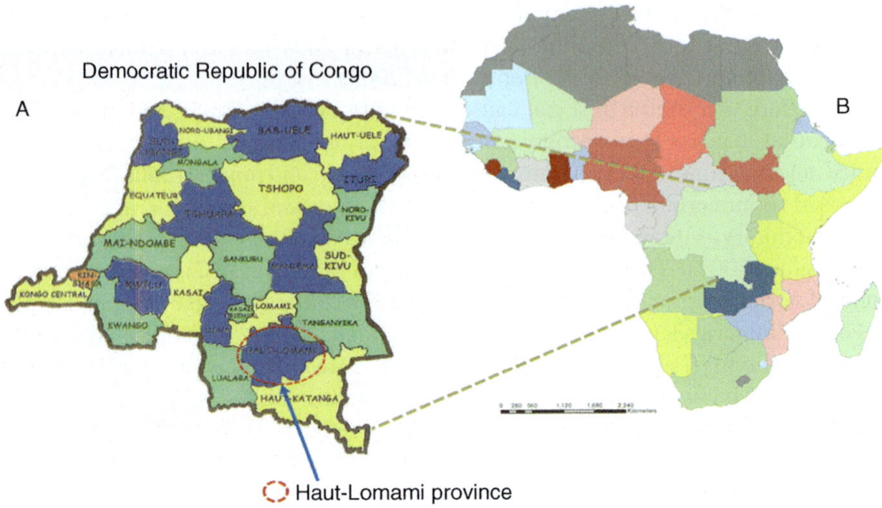

Fig. 5.1 New map of the Democratic Republic of Congo (DRC) (**a**) and map of Africa (**b**). [**a**, image from a co-author (RW: Consultant of DRC National Malaria Program, DRC Ministry of Health); **b**, © 2013 Omumbo et al. Plos One 2013]. (**a**) Shows the location of Haut-Lomami Province (red circle) in DRC, surrounded by four provinces (Lomami, Tanganyika, Haut-Katanga, and Lualaba), whereas (**b**) shows the map of Africa with DRC located at the center

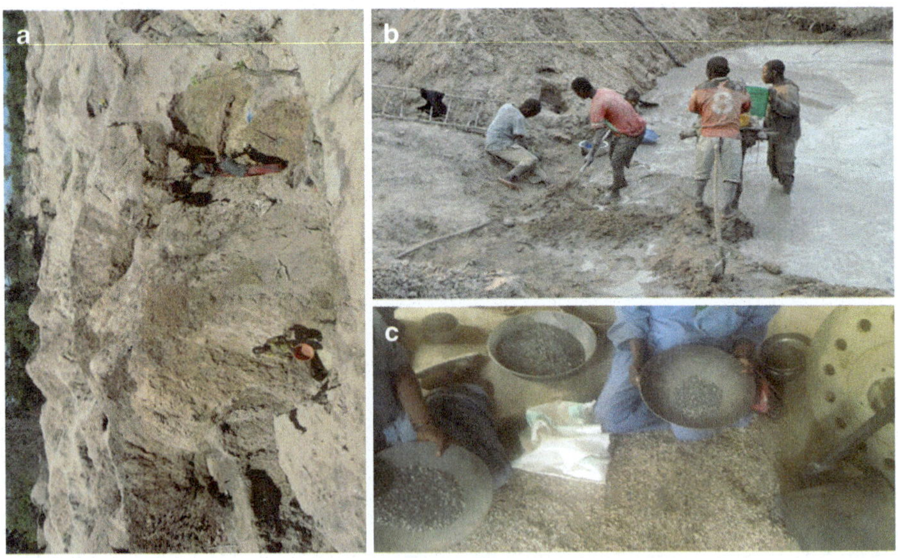

Fig. 5.2 An informal coltan mining site in Lomami province, Democratic Republic of Congo (Photos from authors). This figure shows open-pit coltan mines and miners (**a**, **b**) and samples of manually processed coltan (**c**)

Informal underground and open-pit coltan mining is a risky occupation, with procedures that often expose miners to high dust levels and wet materials (Fig. 5.2). Apart from workstation inspection, a general physical examination was performed (vital signs, weight, height measurement, auscultation); the ambient air quality (PM2.5 and volatile organic compounds or VOC levels) was monitored at each workstation with the use of BRAMC Air Quality Monitor BR-AIR-329 (Shandong, China). In addition, each participant had to answer questionnaires that comprised questions related to the skin and respiratory health. French version of the questionnaires was used. For skin health, six questions related to dermatitis were used; they were extracted from the "Behavioral Risk Factor Surveillance System (BRFSS) state-added dermatitis questions" (St. Louis et al. 2014) and included information on previous dermatitis occurring in the last 12 months and those that occurred previously:

1. "During the past 12 months, have you had dermatitis (itchy, burning, or painful skin) eczema or any other red, inflamed skin rash that you think is related to your work, and have you had similar condition in the past 2 or more years?"
2. "Have you ever seen a doctor or other health professional for your skin condition?"
3. "Have you been told by a doctor or other health professional that your skin condition was probably work-related?"
4. "Do you think your skin condition was probably work-related?"
5. "Did you tell a doctor or health professional that your skin condition was work-related?"
6. "During the past 12 months, did you stop working, change jobs, or make a major change in your work activities, such as taking on lighter duties, because of your skin condition" (St. Louis et al. 2014)?

5.2.2 Ethical Considerations and Statistical Analysis

Each of the study participants provided a signed informed consent form. The study was undertaken in conformity with the Helsinki declaration on the use of humans in research, as revised in 2000. Participation was voluntary, and the study protocol was approved by the ethics committee of the School of Public Health of the University of Lubumbashi, DRC. Photos used in this report are from authors, and permission to use them in this report was obtained. Data were encoded using Excel software; statistical analyses were performed by means of Stata software package version 14 (StataCorp LP, College Station, TX, USA). To compare the study groups (coltan miners and controls), Pearson's chi-square test and Student's *t*-test were performed for categorical and continuous variables related to sociodemographic, occupational, and clinical characteristics, respectively. In addition, a multivariate linear regression analysis was used for continuous variables related to lung function and blood pressure, whereas multiple logistic regression was performed to assess the association between participants' characteristics and dichotomous variables related to respiratory symptoms. p-Values (double-sided) less than 0.05 were considered significant.

5.3 Results and Discussion

5.3.1 *Characteristics of Study Participants and Air Quality in Workplaces*

Data from 199 informal coltan miners and 199 office workers ($N = 398$) were analyzed; they were all males, living in the same town. No statistically significant difference was observed when comparing the age of miners and controls (32.7 ± 8.3 vs. 34.2 ± 9.5) years, respectively). There were more smokers among coltan miners than controls (90.4% vs. 42.2%, respectively; $p < 0.001$). Additionally, regarding daily work duration, a higher proportion of controls worked longer (>8 h) as compared with miners (65.8% vs. 9.5%; $p < 0.001$). When considering working years, no statistically significant difference was noted between the two study groups (Table 5.1). Moreover, field inspections and workstation dust monitoring showed alarming results for coltan mining site. A large majority of miners did not use appropriate personal protective equipment (PPE) to protect their eyes and nose, and any other safety measures (e.g., ventilation) that reduce dust exposure level were in

Table 5.1 Sociodemographic and occupational characteristics of participants

Characteristics	Controls ($n = 199$)	Coltan miners ($n = 199$)	p-value
Age (Mean ± SD)	34.2 ± 9.5	32.7 ± 8.3	0.096
Weight (Mean ± SD)	61.9 ± 11.8	58.4 ± 5.1	**0.045**
Height (Mean ± SD)	163.6 ± 6.9	161.2 ± 7.7	**0.049**
Education level [*n* (%)]			
Low	68 (34.1)	59 (29.6)	–
High	131 (65.8)	140 (70.3)	0.333
Alcohol intake [*n* (%)]			
Yes	79 (39.7)	168 (84.4)	**0.000**
No	120 (60.3)	31 (15.6)	–
Smoking [*n* (%)]			
Yes	84 (42.2)	180 (90.4)	**0.000**
No	115 (57.8)	19 (9.6)	–
Number/cigarettes (Mean ± SD)	4.7 ± 3.2	11.1 ± 5.3	–
Daily work duration [*n* (%)]			
8 h or less	68 (34.1)	180 (90.4)	**0.000**
>8 h	131 (65.8)	19 (9.5)	**–**
Working years [*n* (%)]			
<5 y	69 (34.7)	85 (42.7)	0.100
5 y or more	130 (65.3)	114 (57.3)	–

SD standard deviation, *y* year, *n* number of participants

2A

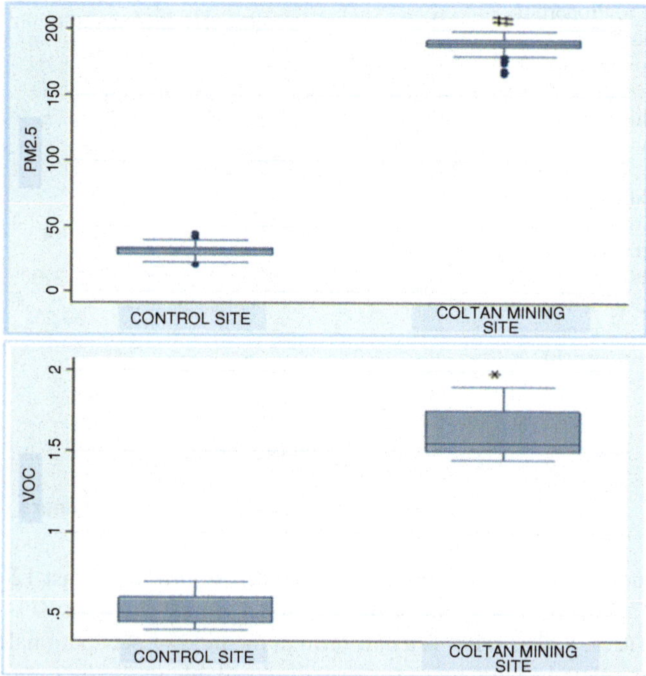

2B

Fig. 5.3 Mean dust (PM2.5, VOC) levels in coltan mining and control settings. *PM2.5* particulate matter; *VOC* volatile organic compounds. This figure shows that higher PM2.5 (**a**) and VOC (**b**) concentrations were detected in coltan miners' workstations as compared with controls' work site

use in coltan processing stations. Furthermore, higher PM2.5 levels were detected in the mining site than in control site (range, 180–210 μg/m^3 vs. 19–44 μg/m^3, respectively; $p < 0.001$); similarly, higher VOC levels were also found in miners' workstations (range, 1.4–2.3 vs. 0.5–0.8, respectively; $p < 0.05$), suggesting that coltan mining settings were hazardous dusty workplace (Fig. 5.3a, b). The PM2.5 levels that were recorded in informal coltan mining setting were very high compared to the exposure limit recommended by the World Health Organization (WHO 2016), 25 μg/m^3 in average.

5.3.2 Proportion of Miners and Controls with Dermatitis in the Last 12-Month Period and Previously (in Their Career and Prior to Last 12 Months)

Figure 5.4 shows the frequency of WRD among coltan miners, as well as the proportion of unexposed office workers (controls) who have developed dermatitis symptoms in the last 12 months and previously. It was observed that dermatitis was

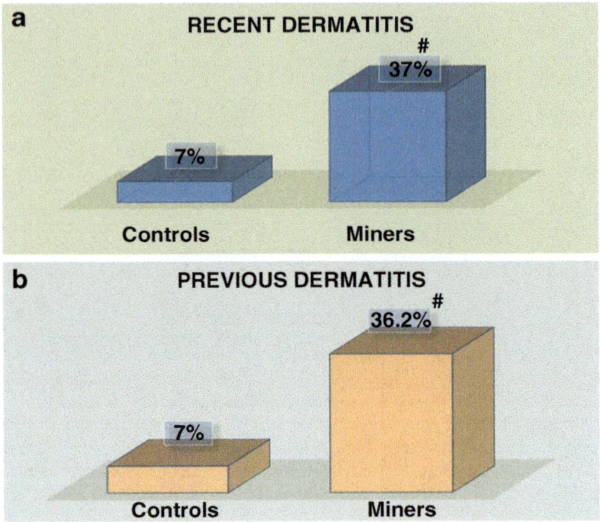

Fig. 5.4 (**a**, **b**) Proportion of coltan miners and controls who developed at least one dermatitis episode in the last 12 months and previously. #, *p*-value less than 0.001. Note that markedly higher proportions of self-reported dermatitis among coltan miners (vs. controls) in the last 12-month period (**a**) (37% vs. 7%) and also before the last year (**b**) (36.2% vs. 7%) were observed

more frequent among coltan miners than controls both in the last 12-month period (37% vs. 7%) (Fig. 5.4a) and in the previous years (36.2% vs. 7%, respectively; $p < 0.001$) (Fig. 5.4b). WRD is a new term in the field of occupational skin diseases; and reports related to this topic are scarcely available in the literature. The proportion of self-reported WRD (36–37%) found in this study is high. Previously, St. Louis et al. (2014) reported a prevalence of self-reported WRD varying from 12.9% and 17.6% in the US working population.

5.3.3 Association Between Miners' Characteristics, Air Quality, and Work-Related Dermatitis

In order to determine coltan miners' characteristics that are associated with the risk of developing WRD, a multiple logistic regression analysis was performed. In the bivariate analysis, it was observed that coltan mining work was strongly associated with "recent dermatitis" (OR = 7.48 ± 2.35; 95% CI, 4.04–13.86; $p < 0.001$) and "previous dermatitis" (OR = 7.42 ± 2.45; 95% CI, 4.23–14.46; $p < 0.001$) (Table 5.2). On the other hand, a multivariate analysis was performed with adjustment for age, height, BMI, and smoking that showed that coltan miners had a 4.88 times risk of developing dermatitis in the last 12-month period (OR = 4.88 ± 1.15; 95% CI, 2.06–11.33; $p < 0.05$) and a 9.48 times higher risk of dermatitis in previous years (OR = 9.48 ± 12.3; 95% CI, 3.74–120.49; $p < 0.005$) (Table 5.2). Furthermore, a correlation analysis between work station dust levels and the occurrence of WRD in coltan miners showed that PM2.5 exposure was positively correlated with recent dermatitis (Rho = 0.35; $p < 0.0001$) and also with previous dermatitis (Rho = 0.37; $p < 0.0001$). In addition, similar findings were observed in regard to work station VOC levels (not shown).

Table 5.2 Association between participants' characteristics (coltan miners vs. controls) and work-related dermatitis

Characteristics	OR	aOR	SE	95% CI	*p*-value
Age	0.99	0.87	0.19	0.56–1.36	0.562
Height	0.84	0.94	0.01	0.91–0.97	0.067
BMI	1.89	0.89	0.03	0.82–0.97	0.078
Previous dermatitis	7.82	9.48	12.32	3.74–12.05	**0.023**
Recent dermatitis	7.49	4.88	1.15	2.06–11.33	**0.047**

OR unadjusted odds ration, *aOR* adjusted odds ratio

In fact, environmental and occupation dust exposures are reported to induce and aggravate dermatitis, especially eczema. A recent report a Korean research team showed that exposure to high concentrations of particulate matters (PM2.5, PM10) was associated with atopic eczema symptoms in Korean children living in industrialized urban area (Oh et al. 2018). One of the reasons is that fine particulates such as PM2.5 easily penetrate the skin (Kimata 2004).

5.4 Conclusion

This is the first study reporting on the skin health of African coltan miners. Worksite investigations in Congolese coltan mining settings revealed striking findings; most miners worked bare hands without appropriate PPE that could protect them against dust. Surprisingly, workstation dust (PM2.5, VOC) levels were tremendously high. This study also revealed high proportion of WRD among coltan miners and that dust exposure was positively associated with dermatitis. Implementation of safety measures and dust control measure that reduce exposure and mitigate the adverse effects of dust (ventilation, water infusion, etc.), and regulation of this informal business by health policymakers should be envisaged to protect the health of miners.

References

Belsito DV. Occupational contact dermatitis: etiology, prevalence, and resultant impairment/disability. J Am Acad Dermatol. 2005;53(2):3030–313.

Sutherland E. Coltan, the Congo and your cell phone. 2011. https://minerals.usgs.gov/minerals/pubs/country/2013/myb3-2013-cg.pdf Accessed 23 Dec 2017.

Donoghue AM. Occupational health hazards in mining: an overview. Occup Med (Lond). 2004;54(5):283–9.

Kabamba NL, Ngatu RN, Kayembe JMN, et al. Silicotuberculosis in African underground miners. Ann Afr Med. 2016;9(2):2218–26.

Kimata H. Exposure to road traffic enhances allergic skin wheal responses and increases plasma neuropeptides and neurotrophins in patients with atopic eczema/dermatitis syndrome. Int J Hyg Environ Health. 2004;207(1):45–9.

Luckhaupt SE, Dahlhamer JM, Ward BW, et al. Prevalence of dermatitis in the working population, United States, 2010 National Health Interview Survey. Am J Ind Med. 2013;56(6):625–34.

Oh I, Lee J, Ahn K, et al. Association between particulate matter concentration and symptoms of atopic dermatitis in children living in an industrial urban area of South Korea. Environ Res. 2018;160:462–8.

Omumbo JA, Noor AM, Fall IS, et al. How well are malaria maps used to design and finance malaria control in Africa? PLoS One. 2013;8(1):e53198.

Poplin GS, Miller HD, Hintz PJ, et al. Dermatitis in the mining industry: incidence, sources, and time loss. Arch Environ Occup Health. 2005;60(2):77–85.

St. Louis T, Ehrlich E, Bunn T, et al. Proportion of dermatitis attributed to work exposures in the working population, United States, 2011 behavioral Risk Factor Surveillance System. Am J Ind Med. 2014;57(6):653–9.

Taylor JS, Amado A. Contact dermatitis and related conditions. Center for Continuing Education Report 2010. 2010. http://www.clevelandclinicmeded.com/medicalpubs/diseasemanagement/dermatology/contact-dermatitis-and-related-conditions/. Accessed 10 Dec 2017.

US Department of Labor. Workplace injuries and illnesses in 2008. 2010. http://www.bls.gov.news.release/pdf/osh.pdf. Accessed 12 Dec 2017.

World Health Organization (WHO). Ambient (outdoor) air quality and health. 2016. http://www.who.int/mediacentre/factsheets/fs313/en/.

Yager T. Mineral industry of Congo (Kinshasa). US Department of Interior. 2016. https://minerals.usgs.gov/minerals/pubs/country/2013/myb3-2013-cg.pdf. Accessed 23 Dec 2017.

Chapter 6
Occupational Cement Dermatitis and Cement Burns

Ngombe Leon-Kabamba, Sakatolo Jean-Baptiste Kakoma, Numbi Oscar-Luboya, Mukanya Pascal-Kimba, Nkulu C. Banza-Lubamba, Nlandu Roger Ngatu, and Benoit Nemery

Abstract Cement is a material with a wide industrial usage and is the leading cause of occupational skin disorders in construction workers. Cutaneous exposure to cement, particularly wet cement, is reported to cause contact dermatitis, contact urticaria, and skin burn. These skin disorders often occur in construction settings; however, they are not extensively reported. A mini-review of literature was conducted; in addition, we present the case of a young African man who developed severe cement burn caused by wet cement when helping a friend to place a concrete floor. The most common skin lesions and symptoms in case of cement dermatitis are erythema, papules, hyperkeratosis, edema, and/or skin thickening, whereas cement burn is mostly characterized by pain, erosion, and even ulcerative lesions. Our cement burn patient was a 23-year-old male Congolese student who presented with multiple wounds all over his body at the admission. The lesions started 7 days earlier, shortly after having helped a friend to place concrete on a construction site. His job had mainly consisted of carrying buckets containing wet concrete. Prior to visiting us at the hospital, he has been applying palm oil on his wounds without untoward effects. The wounds healed after 3 weeks of conservative treatment.

N. Leon-Kabamba, MD., MPH. (✉)
Toxicology and Environment Unit, Department of Public Health, Faculty of Medicine, University of Kamina, Kamina, Congo
e-mail: leonngombe@yahoo.fr

S. J.-B. Kakoma, MD., PhD. · N. Oscar-Luboya, MD.PhD. · M. Pascal-Kimba, MPH., PhD. · N. C. Banza-Lubamba, MD., PhD.
School of Public Health, University of Lubumbashi, Lubumbashi, Congo

N. R. Ngatu, M.D., Ph.D.
Graduate School of Medicine, International University of Health and Welfare (IUHW), Chiba, Japan

Graduate School of Public Health, International University of Health and Welfare (IUHW), Tokyo, Japan

B. Nemery, MD., PhD.
Occupational & Environmental Medicine, Department of Public Health and Primary Care, KU Leuven, Leuven, Belgium

N. R. Ngatu, M. Ikeda (eds.), *Occupational and Environmental Skin Disorders*,
https://doi.org/10.1007/978-981-10-8758-5_6

Keywords Africa · Cement dermatitis · Cement burn · Congo · Construction work

Abbreviations

ACD Allergic contact dermatitis
ICD Irritant contact dermatitis

6.1 Background

6.1.1 Cement Dermatitis in Construction Workers

Cement is a material with a wide industrial usage and is the leading cause of occupational skin disorders in construction workers. Cutaneous exposure to cement, particularly wet cement, is reported to cause contact dermatitis, contact urticaria, and skin burn (Poppe et al. 2013; Behrangi et al. 2014). In Iran, a case-control study was conducted in 2001 among 150 randomly selected factory workers and 150 office workers (controls) in a cement factory. Participants were interviewed, and information on their past dermatological history and employment duration in the current job position was collected. Findings showed a prevalence rate of contact dermatitis of 22% among cement-exposed workers, whereas it was 5% in the control group (Iraji et al. 2006).

Cement can cause abrasive lesions, irritant contact dermatitis (ICD), and also allergic contact dermatitis (ACD) mainly as a reaction to its hexavalent chromate ions. In addition, prolonged skin contact with wet cement can also cause cement burns (alkali burns) due to the cement's high pH that reach 11–13.

6.1.2 Cement Burn and Ulcerative Skin in Construction Workers

Cement is composed of different chemicals such as calcium dioxide (CaO), sulfur dioxide (SO2), silicon dioxide (SiO2), metalloid and metal compounds, etc. When it is mixed with water, calcium hydroxide ($Ca(OH)_2$) is liberated. As a consequence, an increase in alkalinity will occur with a high pH; and in case of prolonged skin contact with wet cement, an alkali burn, with skin erosion or necrosis, may occur (Buckley 1982; Peters 1984, 2001; Poupon et al. 2005; Chung et al. 2007; Wang et al. 2011; Chiriac et al. 2016). Severe cement burns may require hospitalization, surgery, and skin grafting. Cement burns may occur among masons and other construction workers, but other people may also be affected, especially amateurs involved in do-it-yourself. Although cement burns are probably frequent, they are not frequently reported. Moreover, we found no publications of such lesions from Sub-Saharan countries or descriptions of cement burns in people with a dark skin. We present a case of an African man who suffered extensive and severe burns from working casually with cement work (Lewis et al. 2004; Poupon et al. 2005; Chung et al. 2007).

6.2 Case Presentation

A 23-year-old male Congolese student from Katanga area presented with multiple wounds all over his body at his admission at the hospital. The lesions started 7 days earlier, shortly after having helped a friend to place concrete on a construction site. His job had mainly consisted of carrying buckets containing wet concrete. He had done this for about half a day, wearing a T-shirt, without gloves or protective boots. He noticed skin lesions and started feeling pain in the evening after work. The lesions worsened and became so painful that he had not been able to sleep for the past week. To alleviate the pain, he applied palm oil onto the wounds in the evening of the exposure and then twice a day until coming to the hospital; he had also taken ibuprofen (400 mg) twice a day. The persistence of the wounds and pain had motivated him to seek further treatment.

The patient's medical and surgical history was unremarkable; he was not under any medication, and he reported no alcohol intake, tobacco smoking, or drug abuse. He was a student in secondary school (not unusual at this age, in Congo), and has never worked as employee in construction industry. He was in a good general condition, had no fever, and showed no clinical signs of dehydration or anemia. He had pain with multiple skin lesions on various parts of the body (Fig. 6.1), but not on his face. On the left upper and anterior zone of the chest, he had a large ulcer of yellowish appearance and with scattered scabs (Fig. 6.1a). There were similar, but less extensive wounds on his shoulder (Fig. 6.1b) and abdomen (Fig. 6.1c). Smaller yellowish round lesions were also present on both hands (Fig. 6.1d), both knees, the anterolateral sides of both legs, and both feet (Fig. 6.1e).

Although the burned surface was not formally assessed, about 5% of the total body surface area was affected by the lesions, with several being full-thickness wounds. There were no signs of local infection and the draining lymph nodes were not swollen. The following treatment was given: anti-tetanus serum (3000 units), cefotaxim (3 g/day for 10 days), and metronidazole (1 g/day for 10 days). The wounds were treated locally with the application of Dakin's solution (2000 mg of chloramine in 1 liter of water) daily for 12 days. Complete healing of the wounds, without keloid formation, was achieved 19 days after admission (Fig. 6.2).

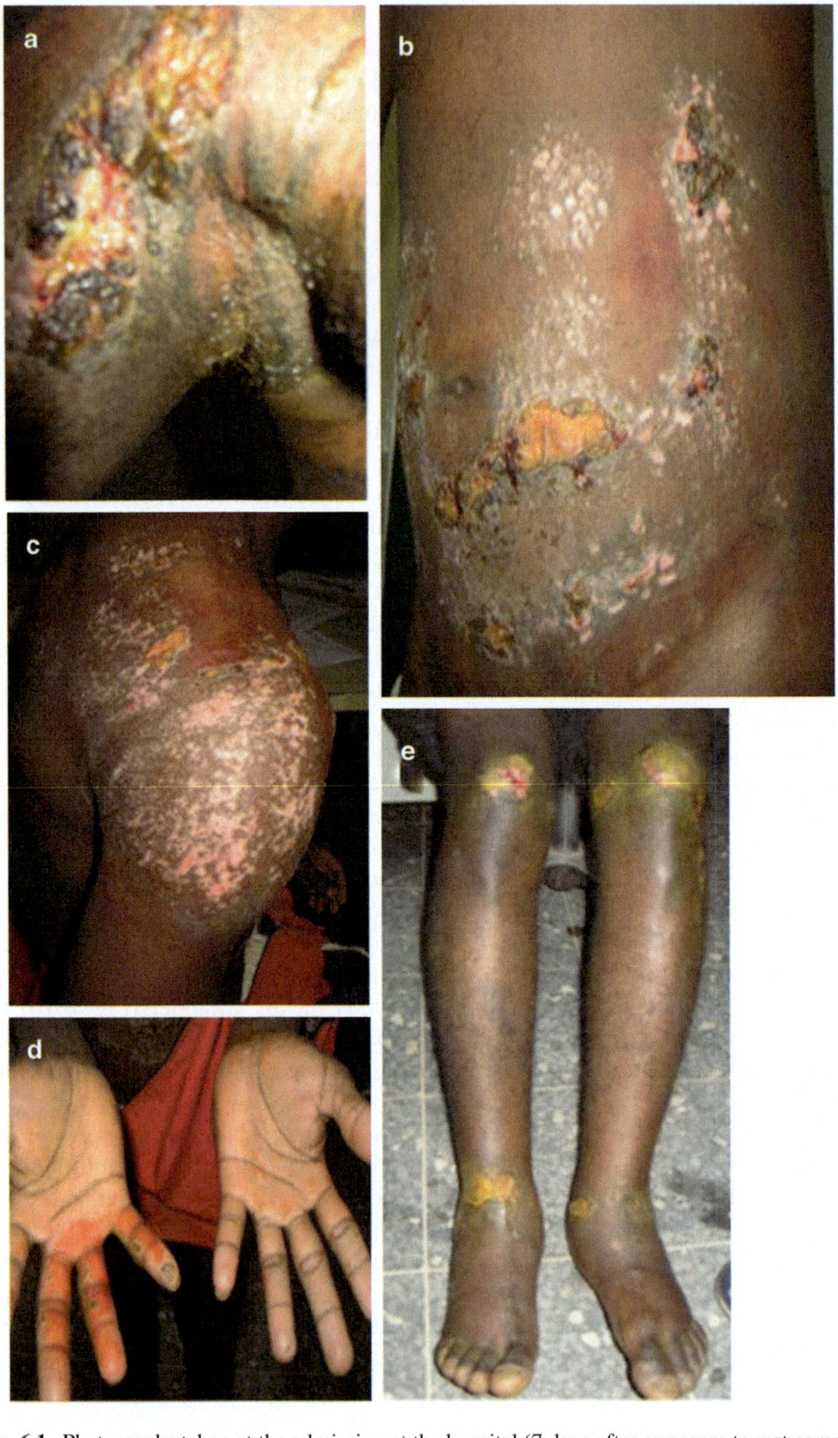

Fig. 6.1 Photographs taken at the admission at the hospital (7 days after exposure to wet cement)

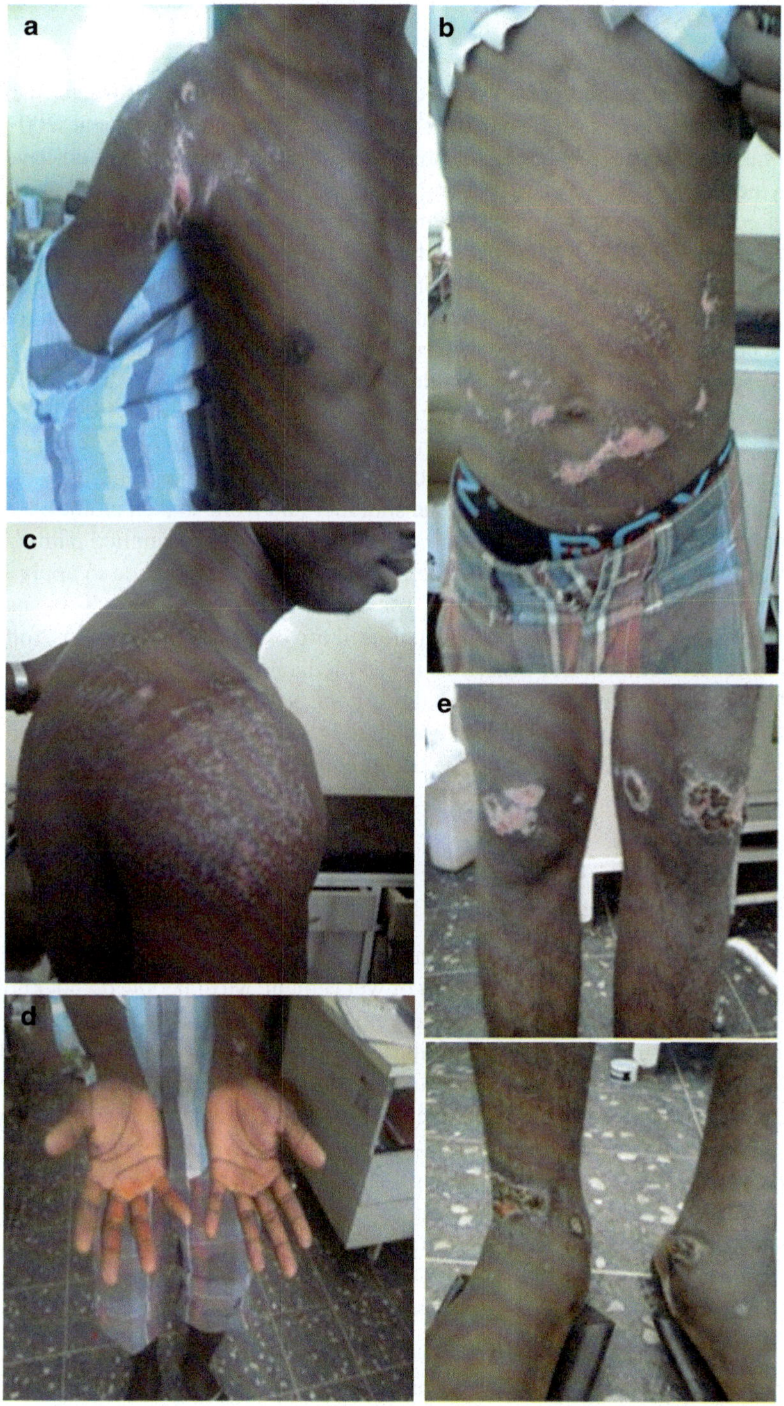

Fig. 6.2 Photographs taken 19 days after presentation, i.e., 26 days after exposure to wet cement

6.3 Discussion

Exposure to wet cement is known to cause occupational skin disorders, including chemical burns (Spoo and Elsner 2001; Poupon et al. 2005; Chung et al. 2007). Our observation confirms that the risk also exists for casual workers and do-it-yourself handymen (Lewis et al. 2004; Chung et al. 2007); due to ignorance and lack of experience, they are even more likely to be exposed to wet cement.

The skin lesions observed on our patient are in lines with what has been described in the literature in regard to skin lesions caused by contact with cement (Spoo and Elsner 2001; Poupon et al. 2005; Chung et al. 2007): rounded lesions with more or less deep ulceration and necrosis. Usually the lesions are located on the fingers, hands, forearms, knees and legs, ankles, or feet, as a result of working with bare hands, kneeling on wet concrete, or getting cement inside boots. However, in our case the localization and very large number of wounds—all four limbs being affected, as well as the trunk—seem to be exceptional. The lesions on the trunk, as in our case, may result from wearing buckets on the shoulder and from soaked clothes.

Our patient simply washed himself after work and he then applied palm oil onto the wounds to in attempt to relieve the pain. It is common practice to apply greasy substances onto burns in the Congo, for example, substances such as snake fat (obtained from boas), honey, but also palm oil are often used. The latter "folk remedy" is not recognized, nor described in the medical literature. However, our anecdotal observation may suggest that palm oil was somewhat effective in alleviating the pain, and it might even have had protected the skin against secondary bacterial infection during the first week before treatment at the hospital.

6.4 Conclusions

The extent and severity of the lesions in the present case can be reasonably attributed to the victim's ignorance of the hazards of wet cement. Most people do not know that cement may cause burns, and they do not realize that severe burns may occur without feeling pain upon contact with the injurious agent. Indeed, unlike acids, alkaline substances do not cause immediate pain. Cement burns should be prevented by adequate product labeling and appropriate warnings—although this does not appear to be very effective (Lewis et al. 2004)—as well as by wearing personal protective equipment (gloves, shoes, and clothing). However, especially in resource-poor settings, on-the-job education and training by peers on how (not) to handle cement are probably the most effective measures to avoid such occupational injuries.

Consent Written informed consent was obtained from the patient for publication of this report and photos.

Competing Interests

The authors declare that they have no competing interests.

Authors' Contributions

N.L.K. provided medical care to patient; N.L.K., N.R.N., and M.I. wrote the successive drafts of the chapter, together with P.K.M.; S.J.B.K., C.B.L.N., B.N., and N.O.L. assisted in writing this chapter and data interpretation. All authors approved the final version of the chapter.

References

Behrangi E, Ansarin H, Fakhim TH, et al. An unusual skin lesion in cement irritant contact dermatitis. J Skin Stem Cell. 2014;1(2):e22012.

Buckley DB. Skin burns due to wet cement. Contact Dermatitis. 1982;8:407–9.

Chiriac A, podoleanu C, Moldovan C, et al. Cement burn: an occupational disease with favorable outcome. Case report. Int Wound J. 2016;13(5):1014–5.

Chung JY, Kowal-Vern A, Latenser BA, et al. Cement-related injuries: review of a series, the National Burn Repository, and the prevailing literature. J Burn Care Res. 2007;28:827–34.

Iraji F, Asilian A, Enshaieh S, et al. Contact dermatitis in cement workers in Isfahan. Indian J Dermatol. 2006;51(1):30–2.

Lewis PM, Ennis O, Kashif A, et al. Wet cement remains a poorly recognized cause of full-thickness skin burns. Injury. 2004;35:982–5.

Peters WJ. Alkali burns from wet cement. Can Med Assoc J. 1984;130(7):902–4.

Poppe H, Poppe LM, Brocker EB, et al. Do-it-yourself cement work: the main cause of severe irritant contact dermatitis requiring hospitalization. Contact Dermatitis. 2013;68(2):111–5.

Poupon M, Caye N, Duteille F, et al. Cement burns: retrospective study of 18 cases and review of the literature. Burns. 2005;31:910–4.

Spoo J, Elsner P. Cement burns: a review 1960-2000. Contact Dermatitis. 2001;45:68–71.

Wang BJ, Wu JD, Sheu SC, et al. Occupational hand dermatitis among workers in Taiwan. J Formosan Med Assoc. 2011;110(12):775–9.

Chapter 7
Alternative Nonsteroidal Therapies for Occupational and Environmental Allergic Skin Disorders

Mitsunori Ikeda

Abstract Topical corticosteroids (TCS) have long been considered as the first-line treatment for allergic skin diseases. Due to corticosteroids-related side effects and their contraindications, the search for alternative anti-inflammatory therapies has proven to be necessary. A mini-review on currently used and potential topical anti-allergic agents that are employed as alternatives to TCS and topical calcineurin inhibitors (TCI) with available clinical reports is done. In case of unsuccessful TCS and TCI therapy in AD patients, a systemic treatment or a phototherapy is often envisaged as next line of defense. For example, phototherapy (broadband UVB (290–320 nm), narrowband UVB (311–313 nm), UVA-1 (340–400 nm), UVA therapy plus 8-methoxypsoralen (PUVA), or full-spectrum light (FSL)) is mainly used to treat severe AD. Other anti-allergic agents currently in use are phosphodiesterase 4 (PDE4) inhibitors (crisaborole and apremilast which reduce the activity of PDE4 enzyme), anti-IgE agents (omalizumab and ligelizumab), IL-4 and IL-13 inhibitors (dupilumab), anti-TNF-α (etanercept, infliximab), and Janus kinase (JAK) inhibitors (e.g., JTE052). Probiotics and other potential anti-allergic plant materials are proposed for AD management; they include biomaterials extracted from Korean red ginseng, African *Vernonia amygdalina* Del., marine algal plants (*Aphanothece sacrum*), etc. Clinicians should consider each patient's history, clinical severity of disease, and the location of skin lesions prior to making a treatment choice.

Keywords Allergic skin disorders · Calcineurin inhibitor · Corticosteroid · Therapy

---

M. Ikeda, M.D., Ph.D.
Graduate School of Nursing, and Wellness & Longevity Center, University of Kochi, Kochi, Japan
e-mail: mikeda@cc.u-kochi.ac.jp

N. R. Ngatu, M. Ikeda (eds.), *Occupational and Environmental Skin Disorders*,
https://doi.org/10.1007/978-981-10-8758-5_7

List of Abbreviations

AZA Azathioprine
CsA Cyclosporin A
IL Interleukin
MMF Mycophenolate mofetil
MTX Methotrexate
TCI Topical calcineurin inhibitor
TCS Topical corticosteroid

7.1 Introduction

Topical corticosteroids (TCS) have long been considered as the first-line treatment for allergic skin diseases. Due to corticosteroid-related side effects and their contraindications, the search for alternative anti-inflammatory therapies has proven to be necessary for the optimum management of eczematous disorders. A few decades ago, topical calcineurin inhibitors (TCI), which are inhibitors of T-lymphocyte activation, have been introduced, mainly in western countries, to address the safety concerns related to local and systemic adverse effects of TCS. They are used as second-line treatment agents for atopic dermatitis (AD). Both TCS and TCI provide good outcomes in terms of pruritus relief, particularly in AD patients. However, the risk of malignancy and the induction of infection on application site have been previously reported. The warning suggests a possible skin absorption of TCI agents that might lead to the induction of systemic side effects such as cancers (Thaci and Salgo 2010; Silverberg et al. 2016). Other immunosuppressive agents, such as cyclosporin A or CsA, azathioprine (AZA), methotrexate (MTX), and mycophenolate mofetil (MMF), have been in use, especially for severe or recalcitrant skin allergic diseases; but similarly, safety concerns relative to the risk of tumor have also been raised. A more recent study by Garritsen et al. (2017) showed a 3% incidence of non-melanoma skin cancer (NMSC), for a NMSC standardized incidence of 13% in immunosuppressive drug-treated AD patients in a sample of 557 patients who underwent oral treatment. We conducted a mini-review on currently used and potential topical anti-allergic agents as alternatives to TCS and TCI with available clinical reports.

7.2 Nonsteroidal Alternative Therapies

Nowadays new therapeutic agents are being introduced either as adjuvant to TCS therapy or therapeutic alternatives to TCS and TCI. In this section, we provide an overview on different nonsteroidal therapies for allergic skin disorders that are supported by clinical investigations.

7.2.1 Phototherapy (UVB, UVA, and Psoralen-UVA or PUVA)

In case of unsuccessful TCS and TCI in the management of AD, a systemic treatment or a phototherapy can be carried out as next line of defense. Currently, phototherapy is mainly reserved for severe AD, and therapeutic modalities include:

- Broadband UVB (290–320 nm) therapy
- Narrowband UVB (311–313 nm) therapy
- UVA-1 (340–400 nm) therapy
- UVA therapy plus 8-methoxypsoralen (PUVA)
- Full-spectrum light (FSL)

However, long-term use is reported to be associated with cutaneous side effects and limitations (Zebda and Paller 2017; Ortiz-Salvador and Perez-Ferriols 2017).

7.2.2 Phosphodiesterase 4 (PDE4) Inhibitors

PDE4 is an enzyme involved in proinflammatory cytokine regulation via the degradation of cyclic adenosine monophosphate (cAMP). In AD patients, the activity of PDE4 is increased; this fact increases the production of several proinflammatory mediators (cytokines and chemokines). Thus, targeting PDE4 will lead to a decrease in the production of the mediators of the allergic inflammation, such as interleukin 4 (IL-4), IL-5, and IL-13 (Saporito and Cohen 2016; Zebda and Paller 2017).

- *Crisaborole* 2% ointment: a US-approved drug for use in children older than 2 years and adults. Recent reports suggest that topical *crisaborole* showed early and sustained improvement in pruritus severity and other AD symptoms' severity as well. As adverse effects, the drug can cause burning or stinging on application site (Zebda and Paller 2017).
- *Apremilast:* the drug is often used in the treatment of plaque psoriasis and psoriatic arthritis, and it is administered orally. Recently, it has attracted the attention of researchers and clinicians as a potential alternative treatment for AD. In an open-label pilot clinical study, Samrao et al. (2012) found that both AD patient groups that received daily 20 mg and 30 mg *apremilast* in 16 patients for 3 months had significantly reduced pruritus and eczema area and severity index (EASI) and improved dermatology life quality index (DLQI). Another 12-week phase 2 open-label clinical trial showed that *apremilast* was well tolerated but minimally effective in reducing EASI score and pruritus in patients with recalcitrant AD or allergic contact dermatitis (ACD) (Volt et al. 2012). Most common side effects were headache and nausea.
- Other PDE4 inhibitors being studied are *roflumilast*, *rolipram*, and *piclamilast*.

7.2.3 Anti-IgE Agents

- *Omalizumab*: it is a humanized monoclonal antibody that is reported to blocks IgE, thus preventing its interaction with its high-affinity receptor (FcεRI) that is present in the membrane of mast cells, dendritic cells, and basophils. The drug is approved for the management of asthma and chronic spontaneous urticarial (Liu et al. 2011). A clinical report from (Kim and colleagues 2013) on the efficacy of omalizumab (fixed schedule of eight cycles of 300 mg administered subcutaneously at 2-week intervals) on ten adult patients (19–35 years of age) with refractory AD showed a relief of AD symptoms in two patients and an improvement in five patients, whereas three patients had no clinical alleviation of their symptoms after a 2-month treatment period.
- Other anti-IgE drugs: ligelizumab is another agent from this group that is being studied. Ligelizumab consists of a humanized IgG1 monoclonal antibody directed against human IgE. However, currently no clinical reports on its safety and effectiveness on allergic skin disorders are available in the literature.

7.2.4 IL-4 and IL-13 Inhibitors

- *Dupilumab*: it is a human monoclonal antibody which blocks IL-4 and IL-13 and currently subject to several clinical trials. For example, a phase II randomized trial for moderate-to-severe adult AD patients showed a relatively rapid improvement in daily 300 mg dupilumab-treated group. In 85% of dupilumab patients, at least 50% of EASI improvement versus 35% in placebo-treated controls after a 12-week treatment period), with a decrease in pruritus severity within the first week of treatment (Beck et al. 2014).

7.2.5 Anti-TNF-α

Tumor necrosis factor alpha (TNF-α) is an inflammatory cytokine known to play a role in the pathogenesis of many chronic inflammatory diseases. Two representatives of this group are of interest for researchers in the field of allergy and other inflammatory disorders:

- *Etanercept and infliximab:* Etanercept is a human recombinant fusion protein, whereas infliximab is a monoclonal antibody that is used as treatment for diseases associated with Th-1 response (Crohn disease, rheumatoid arthritis, psoriasis); both drugs block TNF-α activity by preventing its binding to TNF-a receptor. Up to now, very few case reports have been published that showed contradictory results (Buka et al. 2005; Cassano et al. 2006; Rullan and Murase 2009).

7.2.6 *Janus Kinase (JAK) Inhibitor*

Several inflammatory cytokines elicit their pathophysiologic properties through the JAK-STAT (signal transducer and activator of transcription) signaling pathway, such as IL-4, IL-5, IL-13, and IL-31. Currently, one JAK inhibitor is being studied.

- JTE 052: it is a novel JAK inhibitor developed at Japanese Tobacco, Osaka, that has been reported to inhibit JAK1, JAK2, JAK3, and tyrosine kinase2 (Amano et al. 2015). Previous experiments on animal model of AD have shown very promising results. Additionally, the first report on a randomized controlled clinical trial conducted in 327 adult AD patients was published very recently (Nakagawa et al. 2017), showing clinical effectiveness and good safety profile of all JTE-052 doses tested (varying from 0.25% to 3%), with better effects for 3% JTE052 ointment, as compared to vehicle and 0.1% tacrolimus (positive control).

7.2.7 *Natural Topical Anti-allergic Products and Skin Barrier Enhancer*

- *Probiotics*: their prophylactic effects on AD have been supported by several studies; however, clinical evidence on probiotics' benefice in the management of AD has been lacking. One of the recent systematic reviews and meta-analysis of 13 randomized controlled trials (RCTs) undertaken previously showed good results in terms of SCORAD (scoring of atopic dermatitis) score for some studies and contrasting outcomes for others. Studies with encouraging findings were from Asia, and most of them were related to *Lactobacillus rhamnosus* GG (Huang et al. 2017). Another meta-analysis of RCTs that included eight studies (both preventive and therapeutic studies) showed that probiotics containing mixed strains of bacteria were more effective, particularly when used in subjects aged 1 year or older (Chang et al. 2016).
- *Plant-based anti-allergic agents*: a few number of natural biomaterials from plants have been proved to exert anti-allergic activity in humans. A number of plant materials from the Chinese herbal medicine have been reported to possess anti-allergic property and cases have been reported. However, their safety and effectiveness still need to be assessed in clinical trials with larger samples (Hon et al. 2011). Recent experimental and clinical reports on the anti-allergic effects of other plant-derived biomaterials such as Korean red ginseng (Lee and Son 2011), African *Vernonia amygdalina*, and also sacran, a glycosamino-glycan-like compound from river alga *Aphanothece sacrum* have shown their potential as anti-allergic agents (Ngatu et al. 2012). The two last agents have also demonstrated filaggrin (FLG) and proFLG modulatory activity and skin barrier enhancing property (Ngatu et al. 2014, 2017; Motoyama et al. 2016; Fukushima et al. 2016). Related reports are provided separately in this book.

7.3 Conclusion

Pharmacologic anti-allergic agents such as TCS and TCI are undoubtedly of importance in the management of atopic and contact dermatitis. However, side effects and contraindications related to those drugs make indispensable the finding of alternative therapeutic agents. Currently, there are clinical evidence of the safety and effectiveness of other anti-inflammatory and anti-allergic agents such as JAK inhibitor JTE-052, IL-4 and IL-13 inhibitor dupilumab, PDE4 inhibitor apremilast, and some plant-based biomaterials that have a potential to serve as adjuvant and/or therapeutic alternatives to TCS and TCI in the management of cutaneous allergic disorders.

References

Amano W, Nakajima S, Kunugi H, et al. The Janus kinase inhibitor JTE-052 improves skin barrier function through suppressing signal transducer and activator of transcription 3 signaling. J Allergy Clin Immunol. 2015;136(3):667–677.e7.

Beck LA, Thaci D, Hamilton JD, et al. Dupilumab treatment in adults with moderate-to-severe atopic dermatitis. N Engl J Med. 2014;371(2):130–9.

Buka RL, Resh B, Roberts B, et al. Etanercept minimally effective in 2 children with atopic dermatitis. J Am Acad Dermatol. 2005;53:358–9.

Cassano N, Loconsole F, Coviello C, et al. Infliximab in recalcitrant severe atopic eczema associated with contact allergy. Int J Immunolpathol Pharmacol. 2006;19(1):237–40.

Chang YS, Trivedi MK, Jha A, et al. Synbiotics for prevention and treatment of atopic dermatitis: a meta-analysis of randomized clinical trials. JAMA Pediatr. 2016;170(3):236–42.

Fukushima S, Motoyama K, Tanida Y. Clinical evaluation of novel natural polysaccharides sacran as a skincare material for atopic dermatitis patients. Journal of Cosmetics, Dermatological Sciences and Applications. 2016;6:9–18.

Garritsen FM, van der Schaft J, van der Reek JM, et al. Risk of non-melanoma skin cancer in patients with atopic dermatitis treated with oral immunosuppressive drugs. Acta Derm Venereal. 2017;97(6):724–30.

Huang R, Huacheng N, Shen M, et al. Probiotics for the treatment of atopic dermatitis in children: a systematic review and meta-analysis of randomized controlled trials. Front Cell Infect Microbiol. 2017;7:392.

Kim DH, Park KY, Kim BJ, et al. Anti-immunoglobulin E in the treatment of refractory atopic dermatitis. Clin Exp Dermatol. 2013;38(5):496–500.

Lee KG, Son SW. Efficacy of Korean red ginseng in the treatment of atopic dermatitis. J Ginseng Res. 2011;35(2):149–54.

Liu FT, Goodarzi H, Chen HY. IgE, mast cells, and eosinophils in atopic dermatitis. Clin Rev Allergy Immunol. 2011;41:298–310.

Motoyama K, Tanida Y, Hata K, et al. Anti-inflammatory effects of novel polysaccharide sacran extracted from Cyanobacterium aphanothece sacrum in various inflammatory animal models. Biol Pharm Bull. 2016;39(7):1172–8.

Nakagawa H, Nemoto O, Igarashi A, et al. Efficacy and safety of topical JTE-052, a Janus kinase inhibitor, in Japanese adult patients with moderate-to-severe atopic dermatitis: a phase 2, multicentre, randomized, vehicle-controlled clinical study. Br J Dermatol. 2017;178:424–32. https://doi.org/10.1111/bjd.16014.

Ngatu NR, Okajima MK, Yokogawa M, et al. Anti-allergic effects of Vernonia amygdalina leaf extracts in hapten-induced atopic dermatitis-like disease in mice. Allergol Int. 2012;61(4):597–607.

Ngatu NR, Hirota R, Okajima MK, et al. Efficacy of leaf extracts of Vernonia amygdalina Del. from central Africa on atopic eczema. Ann Phytomed. 2014;3(1):43–9.

Ngatu NR, Motoyama K, Nishimura Y, et al. Anti-allergic and profilaggrin (ProFLG)-mRNA expression modulatory effects of sacran. Int J Biol Macromol. 2017;105(Pt 2):1532–8.

Ortiz-Salvador JM, Perez-Ferriols A. Phototherapy in atopic dermatitis. Adv Exp Med Biol. 2017;996:279–86.

Rullan P, Murase J. Two cases of chronic atopic dermatitis treated with soluble tumor necrosis factor receptor therapy. J Drug Dermatol. 2009;8:873–6.

Samrao A, Berry TM, Goreshi R, et al. A pilot study of an oral phosphodiesterase inhibitor (apremilast) for atopic dermatitis in adults. Arch Dermatol. 2012;148(8):890–7.

Saporito RC, Cohen DJ. Apremilast use for moderate-to-severe atopic dermatitis in pediatric patients. Case Rep Dermatol. 2016;8:1709.184.

Silverberg JI, Nelson DB, Yosipovitch G. Addressing treatment challenges in atopic dermatitis with novel topical therapies. J Dermatol Treat. 2016;27(6):568–76.

Thaci D, Salgo R. Malignancy concerns of topical calcineurin inhibitors for atopic dermatitis: facts andcontroversies. Clin Dermatol. 2010;28(1):52–6.

Volt EM, Au SC, Dumont N, et al. A phase 2, open-label, investigator-initiated study to evaluate the safety and efficacy of apremilast in subjects with recalcitrant allergic contact dermatitis or atopic dermatitis. J Drugs Dermatol. 2012;11(3):341–6.

Zebda R, Paller AS. Phosphodiesterase 4 (PDE4) inhibitors. J Am Acad Dermatol. 2017;78(3S1):S43–52.

Chapter 8
Sacran: Novel Sulfated Polysaccharide as Anti-Allergic Skincare Biomaterial for Atopic Dermatitis

Keiichi Motoyama, Taishi Higashi, Nlandu Roger Ngatu, Maiko Kaneko Okajima, Yasumitsu Nishimura, Hidetoshi Arima, and Tatsuo Kaneko

Abstract Atopic dermatitis (AD) is a skin disease characterized by inflammation, pruritus, and chronic or relapsing eczematous lesions. AD negatively affects quality of life for both patients with AD and their caregivers. We conducted a review of the literature on the beneficial effects of sacran on allergic skin diseases using published biochemical, experimental, and clinical reports. Sacran is a marine alga-derived glycosaminoglycan-like sulfated polysaccharide; it is extracted from the Japanese indigenous cyanobacterium *Aphanothece sacrum*, which is mass-aquacultured in rivers with a high ionic concentration and possesses plenty of a jelly-like extracellular matrix with high water content (97.5–98.3%). Sacran is a heteropolysaccharide composed of various sugar residues (galactose, glucose, mannose, xylose, rhamnose, fucose, galacturonic acid, and glucuronic acid) and contains traces of alanine, galactosamine, uronic acids (these uronic acids have yet to be determined chemically), and muramic acid; 11% of the monosaccharides contain a sulfate group, and 22% of them contain a carboxyl group. Our previous studies have shown that topical sacran markedly reduced transepidermal water loss (TEWL) in dry skin human subjects and displayed similar anti-allergic effects than *hydrocortisone* and

K. Motoyama, Ph.D. (✉) · T. Higashi, PhD. · H. Arima, PhD.
Graduate School of Pharmaceutical Sciences, Kumamoto University, Kumamoto, Japan
e-mail: motoyama@kumamoto-u.ac.jp

N. R. Ngatu, M.D., Ph.D.
Graduate School of Medicine, International University of Health and Welfare (IUHW), Chiba, Japan

Graduate School of Public Health, International University of Health and Welfare (IUHW), Tokyo, Japan

M. K. Okajima, PhD. · T. Kaneko, PhD.
School of Materials Science, Japan Advanced Institute of Science and Technology (JAIST), Nomi, Japan

Y. Nishimura, PhD.
Department of Hygiene, Kawasaki Medical School, Kurashiki, Japan

N. R. Ngatu, M. Ikeda (eds.), *Occupational and Environmental Skin Disorders*,
https://doi.org/10.1007/978-981-10-8758-5_8

tacrolimus in animal experiments. Moreover, our recent clinical studies showed that topical sacran significantly decreased the severity of AD skin lesions, itch, and sleep disorder in AD patients within 4 weeks of topical treatment. Taken together, findings from these studies suggest that topical sacran may serve as an alternative adjuvant and therapeutic anti-allergic agent.

Keywords Allergy · Atopic dermatitis · Cytokine · Filaggrin · Sacran · Skin barrier · Transepidermal water loss

Abbreviations

AD Atopic dermatitis
CD Cluster of differentiation
CS Chondroitin sulfate
DNFB 2,4-Dinitro-1-fluorobenzene
FLG Filaggrin
IFN-γ Interferon gamma
IL Interleukin
MCP-1 Monocyte chemoattractant protein-1
PD Prednisolone
TEWL Transepidermal water loss
TNCB 2,4,6-Trinitrochlorobenzene
TNF-α Tumor necrosis factor alpha

8.1 Introduction

8.1.1 Brief Overview on Atopic Dermatitis and Its Management Challenge

Atopic dermatitis (AD) is a skin disease characterized by inflammation, pruritus, and chronic or relapsing eczematous lesions. AD negatively affects quality of life for both patients with AD and their caregivers. Management of AD focuses on maintaining the skin barrier and is recommended by medical societies worldwide. Use of mild, appropriately formulated emollients may provide benefits without interfering with skin barrier function. However, emollients alone may not control eczema or aspects of this skin disorder, especially in severe cases. Therefore, anti-inflammatory and immunomodulatory therapies may be necessary for moderate-to-severe AD until symptom resolution on the skin (e.g., lesions, patches of dryness, or areas that are prone to flare). Nowadays, corticosteroids are commonly administered to reduce the inflammation. However, they can frequently cause a set of serious adverse effects (Hengge et al. 2006; Schoepe et al. 2006). Hence, great efforts have been devoted toward the discovery of new and safe anti-inflammatory drugs.

Recently, numerous beneficial effects of natural polysaccharides have been demonstrated on human health to exhibit a spectrum of biological activities such as antioxidant, antitumor, and anti-inflammatory (Ananthi et al. 2010; Averbeck et al. 2007; Yanase et al. 2009). For example, the heparan sulfate on the surface of all adherent cells modulates the actions of a large number of extracellular ligands (Bernfield et al. 1999). Kawashima et al. reported that oversulfated chondroitin/dermatan sulfate chains are important in selectin and/or chemokine-mediated cellular responses (Kawashima et al. 2002). In addition, hyaluronan alternatively participates in leukocyte recruitment via interaction with CD44 while activating various inflammatory cells, such as macrophages, through CD44-dependent signaling (Taylor and Gallo 2006). Therefore, the field of polysaccharide biology provides new clues and explanations of the process of inflammation and suggests new therapeutic approaches.

8.1.2 Sacran: Chemical Composition, Structure, and Biological Properties

Recently, ampholytic sulfated polysaccharide sacran has attracted a particular attention. It is extracted from the Japanese indigenous cyanobacterium *Aphanothece sacrum*, which is mass-aquacultured in rivers with a high ionic concentration and possesses plenty of a jelly-like extracellular matrix with high water content (97.5–98.3%) (Okajima et al. 2008, 2009a, b and 2010a, b). Sacran is a heteropolysaccharide composed of sugar residues (galactose, glucose, mannose, xylose, rhamnose, fucose, galacturonic acid, and glucuronic acid) and contains traces of alanine, galactosamine, uronic acids (these uronic acids have yet to be determined chemically), and muramic acid; 11% of monosaccharides contain a sulfate group whose 22% contain a carboxyl group (Fig. 8.1).

Sacran is reported to be a supergiant molecule with extremely high molecular weight (1.6×10^7 g/mol) and surprising length (more than 8 μm). The safety of sacran as a biomaterial could be attributed to the long-term usage of *A. sacrum* by inhabitants of the Kyushu region in Japan as a functional food to ameliorate allergic tendency and gastroenteritis.

8.2 Clinical Anti-Allergic Effects of Sacran

Previously, we revealed that sacran has anti-inflammatory effects on 2,4,6-trinitrochlorobenzene (TNCB)-induced AD model mice. In experimental studies, we have found that topical sacran prevented the development of AD-like skin lesions in hapten-challenged NC/Nga mice and also alleviated skin symptoms in allergic mice as efficiently as did topical *hydrocortisone* (Fig. 8.2a–c) (Ngatu et al. 2012, 2016). Additionally, a case study report showed that topical sacran improved AD and contact allergy skin lesions in patients with chronic condition

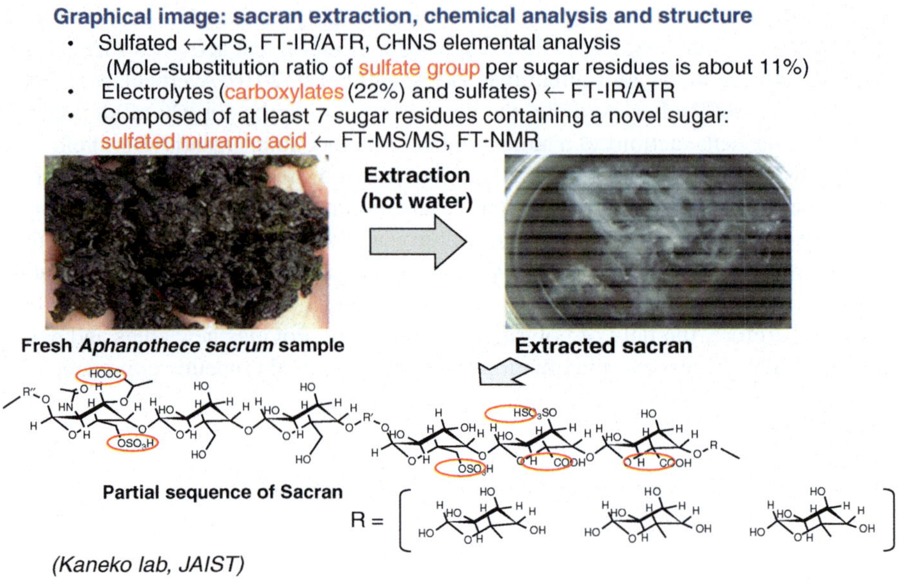

Fig. 8.1 Graphical image of river alga Aphanothece sacrum and hot water extracted sacran and its chemical composition and structure (Image prepared by authors) (Kaneko Lab JAIST)

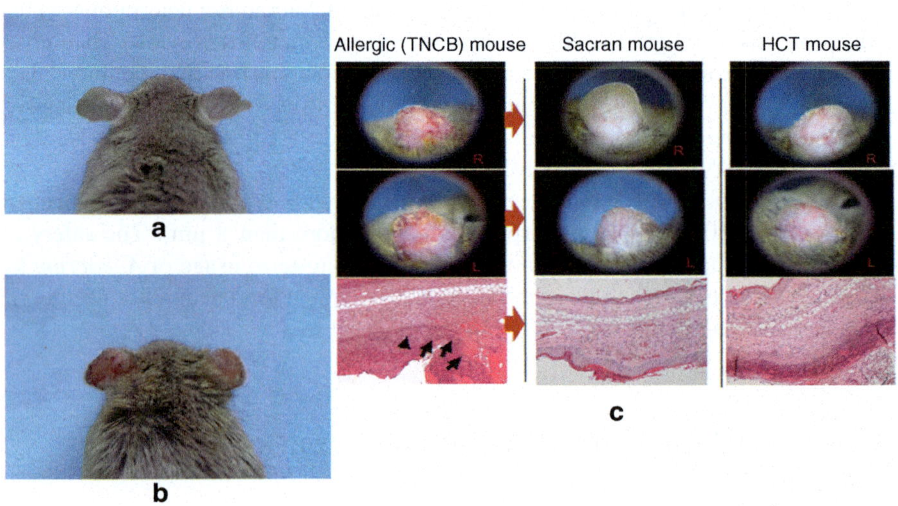

Fig. 8.2 (**a**–**c**) Normal (**a**), diseased mice (**b**), and macroscopic and histologic images (**c**) of mice. [Images from Authors Article and Permission Obtained from Editors; ©2016 Ngatu Roger Nlandu, Attribution 4.0 International (CC BY 4.0)]. *HCT* hydrocortisone, *TNCB* 2,4,6-Trinitrochlorobenze. The figure shows normal mouse ears (**a**) and severe eczematous lesions (edema, erythema, excoriation and scaling) on the right and left ears of the allergic mouse (TNCB) (**b**). However, these processes were markedly reduced in sacran and hydrocortisone (HCT)-treated mice (**c**). Similarly, histologic examination showed intense hemorrhage and cell infiltration in TNCB mouse but mild-to-moderate changes in sacran- and HCT-treated mice

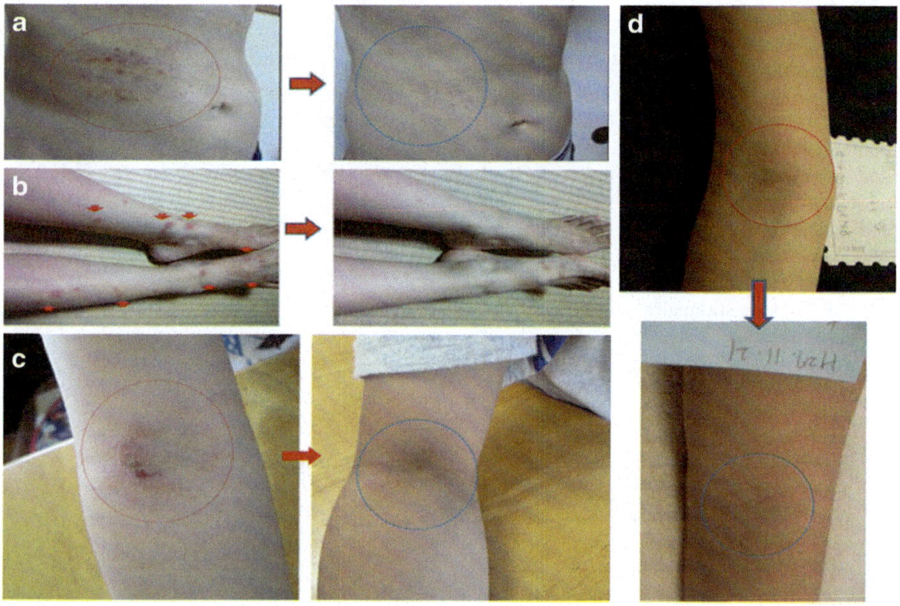

Fig. 8.3 (**a**–**d**) Chronic and recalcitrant allergic skin lesions in an adult atopic patient (**a**), erythematous lesions with itch and burning feeling in a 33-year-old female office worker (**b**) who developed contact hypersensitivity after skin contact with a wild plant in a forest (Ngatu et al. 2015), an 8-year-old girl with atopic dermatitis (**c**), and an 11-year-old girl with chronic atopic dermatitis (**d**). After 1 (patient B) to 3 (patients A, C, and D) weeks of treatment with topical 1% sacran, patients had an improvement of Dermatology Life Quality Index (DLQI) and reduction of total disease severity score. None of the four patients complained of adverse effect that could be induced by the treatment. [Images **a**, **b**: ©Annals Phytomed; images **c**, **d** from the authors]

(Ngatu et al. 2015) (Fig. 8.3a–d). Sacran could relieve pruritus and scaly and erythematous lesions in those patients. Moreover, treatment with sacran did not induce any adverse effects.

Given that no comparative clinical trial has been reported, we investigated the anti-allergic effects of topical application of sacran on AD in the clinical study. In addition, in order to gain insight into the mechanism of its therapeutic effects, we evaluated the potential of sacran as an anti-inflammatory agent in 2,4-dinitro-1-fluorobenzene (DNFB)-induced AD model mice. Figure 3 shows cases of AD (Fig.8.3a–c–d) and environmental CD (Fig.8.3b) patients who have been treated with topical sacran. Improvement of skin symptoms was noted in the second to fourth week of treatment. The beneficial effects of topical sacran on the severity of AD skin lesions and symptoms were evaluated by patients themselves based on questionnaire (13 questions) results. Mean improvement score less than 2 indicates an exacerbation of AD, whereas a score higher than 2 indicates an improvement of patient's skin status.

Almost all of the skin health improvement scores of patients treated with sacran solution were higher than 2 (Fig. 8.4), suggesting an alleviation of AD skin lesions or an improvement of patient condition. In addition, the scores of sleep disorder and

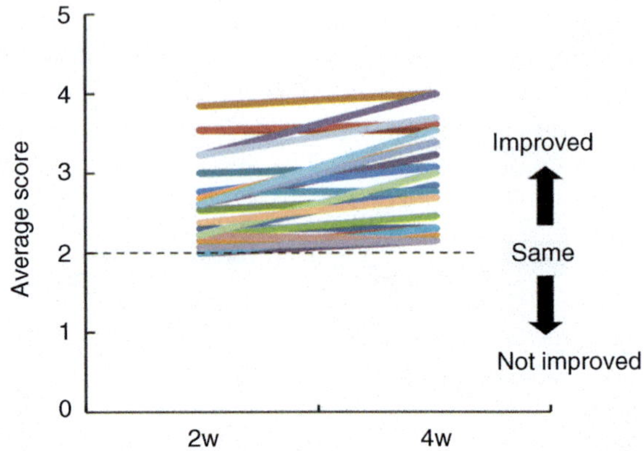

Fig. 8.4 Atopic dermatitis patient self-evaluation of skin status improvement score. Sacran solution was applied for 4 weeks in 25 patients with AD. After 2 and 4 weeks, patients treated with sacran solution self-evaluated the severity of AD symptoms by answering an auto-administered questionnaire (Fukushima et al. 2016)

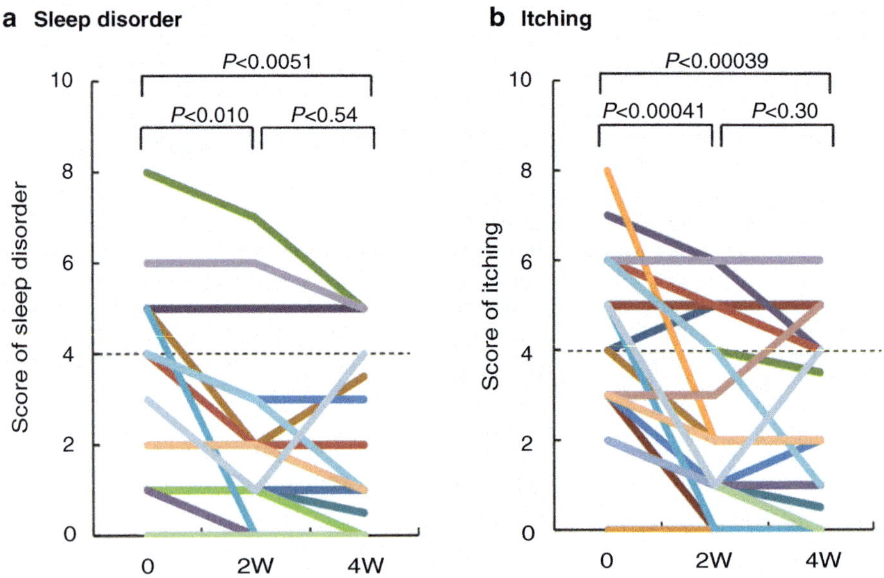

Fig. 8.5 Effect of topical sacran on scores of sleep disorder (**a**) and itch (**b**) in patients with AD (Fukushima et al. 2016) (with the courtesy of J Cosmetics Dermatol Sci Appl editors). Sacran solution was applied for 4 weeks in 25 patients with AD. After 2 and 4 weeks, patients treated with sacran solution self-evaluated the score of sleep disorder and itch

itch tended to decrease during the 4-week sacran treatment with significant differences as compared with baseline scores (Fig. 8.5). Taken together, these results suggest that sacran-treated patients had their AD alleviated.

Based on the dermatologist analysis, the area of rash on the face of AD patients was significantly reduced (Fig. 8.6a). In addition, the total score of rash was also lowered by topical application of sacran within 4 weeks of treatment. Taken together, these findings suggest that sacran has a potential to alleviate AD skin lesions and symptoms (Fig. 8.6b). On the other hand, dry itchy skin worsens the severity of AD

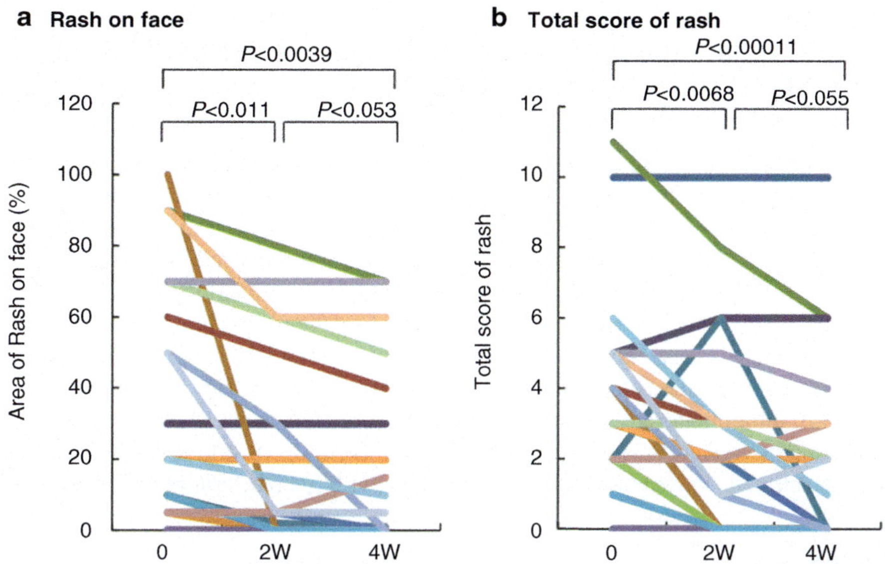

Fig. 8.6 Effect of sacran on area of rash on face (**a**) and total score of rash (**b**) in patients with AD. Sacran was applied for 4 weeks in 25 patients with AD. After 2 and 4 weeks, the medical doctors diagnosed the rash of patients (Fukushima et al. 2016)

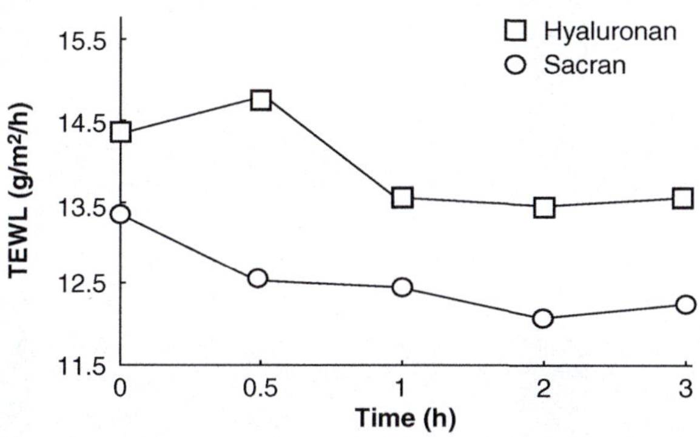

Fig. 8.7 Effects of sacran on transepidermal water loss (TEWL) (Fukushima et al. 2016). TEWL was determined by a VapoMeter Wireless SWL4. Measurements were undertaken after a 20-min rest period. Three measurements were performed on the bony areas of the upper cheek of left and right sides. Each value represents the mean ± S.E. of 10 experiments

and is associated with the increase in scratching behavior (Jin et al. 2009). Next, we therefore investigated the effects of topical application of sacran on TEWL in human subjects with dry skin (Fig. 8.7). It was observed that sacran markedly reduced TEWL as compared with hyaluronan, a well-known polysaccharide that is reported to improve skin moisture and exert skin barrier repair activity (Gu et al. 2010; Ngatu et al. 2012). Thereby, these results suggest that sacran can improve the skin barrier function, thus displaying skin repair activity in AD patients.

8.3 Effects of Topical Sacran on mRNA Levels of Inflammatory Markers in Immature Dermal Skin Model Stimulated with DNFB

The itchy skin elicits scratching behavior, leading to mechanical skin injury and the release of various inflammatory cytokines or chemokines (Homey et al. 2006; Yamashita et al. 2009). Therefore, we examined the effect of sacran on inflammatory cytokine and chemokine mRNA levels in immature dermal skin model stimulated with DNFB. Here, we used immature dermal skin model (Toyobo, Co., Ltd., Osaka, Japan) which simulated the skin of AD patients having low skin barrier function. DNFB was a chemical antigen to evoke contact hypersensitivity reaction and was widely used as an inducer of AD. After treatment with DNFB and sacran for 24 h, inflammatory cytokine and chemokine mRNA levels were determined by real-time PCR. As shown in Fig. 8.8, MCP-1, TNF-α, IL-1β, and IL-6 mRNAs were significantly downregulated by the treatment with sacran, compared to those of

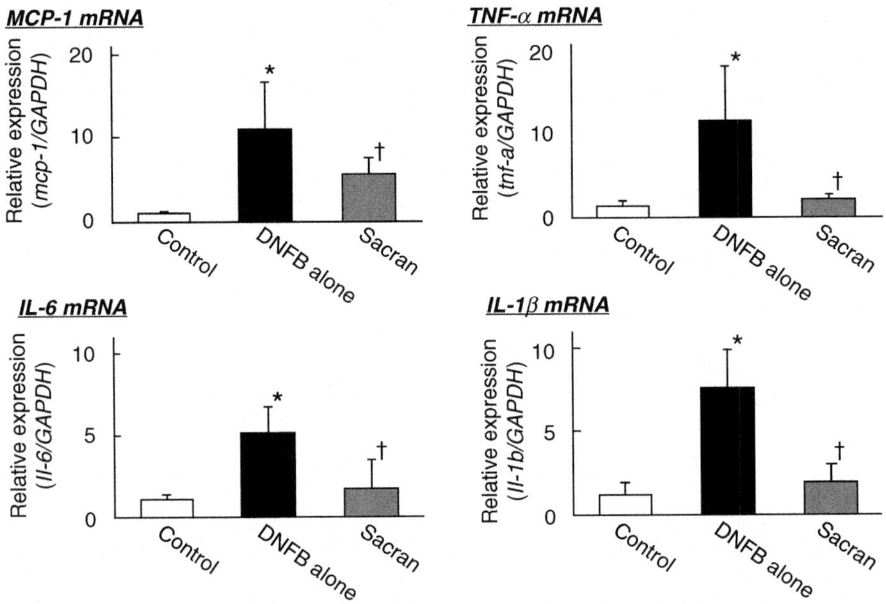

Fig. 8.8 Effects of sacran on mRNA levels in immature dermal skin model after treatment with sacran and DNFB for 24 h (Fukushima et al. 2016). *DNFB* 2,4-dinitro-1-fluorobenzene, *IL* interleukin, *MCP-1* monocyte chemoattractant protein-1, *mRNA* messenger ribonucleic acid, *TNF-α* tumor necrosis factor alpha. A three-dimensional cultured human skin, immature dermal skin model, was incubated with assay medium for 24 h, and then sacran and DNFB were treated for 24 h. The concentrations of sacran and DNFB were 0.05% (w/v) and 0.01% (w/v), respectively. After washing twice with PBS to remove the sample, total RNA was extracted by TRIzol® reagent and then the mRNA levels were determined by real-time PCR. Each value represents the mean ± S.E. of 3 experiments. $^{*}p < 0.05$, compared with control; $^{\dagger}p < 0.05$, compared with DNFB alone

DNFB alone. These results suggest that sacran may have the potential to reduce inflammatory cytokine and chemokine mRNA levels in the skin of AD.

To demonstrate the anti-inflammatory activity of sacran, it is extremely important to investigate whether sacran penetrates into the skin or not. Therefore, we examined the skin penetration of sacran in mature and immature dermal skin for 24 h. As a result, biotinylated sacran (0.05% (w/v)) penetrated the dermis in immature dermal skin model, but not in the mature dermal skin model, simulating the skin of healthy human having rigid skin barrier function (data not shown). This result suggested that sacran can penetrate into AD skin which has impaired barrier function.

8.4 Inhibitory Effects of Sacran Solution on *β-Hexosaminidase* Release

β-Hexosaminidase released from activated mast cells is responsible for the allergic inflammatory responses associated with disease states of AD. Therefore, to examine the anti-allergic activity of sacran, we evaluated the inhibitory effect of sacran on *β-hexosaminidase* release in RBL-2H3 cells, which is now known to be an analog of rat mucosal mast cells (Seldin et al. 1985). As shown in Fig. 8.9, a sacran significantly lowered *β-hexosaminidase* release to 70%, compared to control. These results suggest that a sacran can inhibit the allergic inflammatory responses.

The anti-inflammatory effects displayed by sacran, a unique cyanobacteria-derived glycosaminoglycanoid, could be related to the similarity of its chemical structure to that of glycosaminoglycans, sulfated polysaccharides, which possess numerous bioactivities including an anti-inflammatory effect (Kuschert et al. 1999; Parish 2006; Park et al. 2011; Volpi 2006; Yamada and Sugahara 2008). The high sulfate and carboxyl group content of glycosaminoglycans permits them to interact with a wide range of proteins, enzymes, cytokines, chemokines, lipoproteins, and

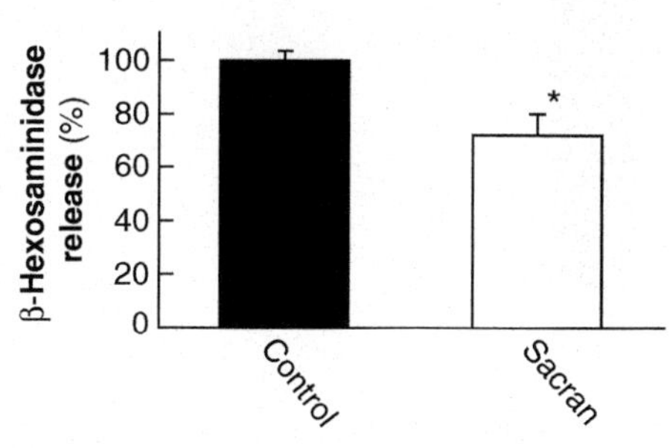

Fig. 8.9 Effect of sacran on β-hexosaminidase release from RBL-2H3 cells. RBL-2H3 cells (2.5×10^5 cells/well) were incubated for 2 h with 500 μL of anti DNP-IgE solution. After washing twice with MT buffer, the cells were incubated in the presence or absence of sacran for 10 min. After adding 10 μL of DNP-HSA solution, the cells were incubated for 30 min. β-Hexosaminidase release (%) = 100 × S/(S + CL); *S* absorbance of supernatant, *CL* absorbance of cell lysate. Each value represents the mean ± S.E. of 3 experiments. *$p < 0.05$, compared with control

adhesion molecules (Bernfield et al. 1999; Kawashima et al. 2002; Taylor and Gallo 2006; Salmivirta et al. 1996). Also, Ngatu et al. reported that epicutaneous application of sacran to 2,4,6-trinitrochlorobenzene-induced NC/Nga mice significantly inhibited the development of AD skin lesions and decreased the number of scratching behavior episodes by improving the stability, elasticity, and hydration of skin barrier as well as inhibiting the production of Th2 cytokines (IL-4, IL-5), Th1 cytokines (TNF-α, IFN-γ and inflammatory chemokines such as MCP-1 and eotaxin, thus inhibiting IgE and eosinophilic infiltration in mice (Ngatu et al. 2012). These sacran properties are not common to sulfated polysaccharides.

8.5 Effect of Sacran Solution on TNF-α and COX-2 mRNA Levels in Macrophages Stimulated with PMA

PMA, a specific activator of protein kinase C (PKC), induces suitable inflammatory responses. Next, to examine whether a sacran can inhibit inflammatory responses in macrophages, we investigated the effect of sacran on the mRNA expression levels of TNF-α and COX-2 in RAW264.7 cells stimulated with PMA. The results showed that 0.05% (w/v) sacran solution significantly suppressed the mRNA expression of TNF-α and COX-2 in macrophages, compared with PMA alone (Fig. 8.10). These results indicate that sacran can reduce the inflammatory responses in macrophages.

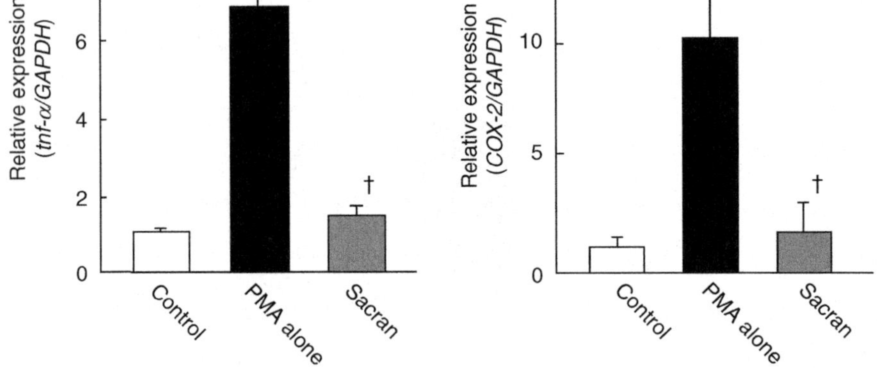

Fig. 8.10 Effect of sacran on TNF-a and COX-2 mRNA levels in RAW264.7 cells stimulated with PMA. RAW264.7 cells (5×10^5 cells/well) were incubated for 24 h. Cells were washed once with PBS, and then incubated with 500 μL of medium containing PMA in the presence or absence of sacran for 2 h. After washing twice with, total RNA was extracted by TRIzol® reagent, and then the mRNA levels were determined by real-time PCR. Each value represents the mean ± S.E. of 8–12 experiments. $*p < 0.05$, compared with control; $\dagger p < 0.05$, compared with PMA alone

8.6 Conclusion

In the present report, we revealed that topical application of sacran displayed anti-allergic effects on hapten-induced AD-like skin disease in mice and also in AD patients. In addition, in experiments exploring the immunomodulatory activity of sacran, it was observed that treatment with sacran reduced TEWL and improved water retention in the skin, inhibited mast cell degranulation, and reduced the production of inflammatory markers (total IgE, TNF-α, COX-2, MCP-1, IL-6, IL-1β, etc.) and upregulated proFLG-mRNA expression.

What is known about the pathogenesis of AD is that the breakdown of the skin barrier results in an increased TEWL, the reduction of skin hydration, and an increased antigen presentation by Langerhans cells (LC) initiating inflammation (Hanifin 2009; Visscher et al. 2015).

In fact, the disruption of skin barrier activates keratinocytes and induces the production of T cells attracting chemokines and cytokines which mediate the innate immune reactions (activation of LC, and also activation of Th2, Th22 cascade with the resulting release of Th2, Th1, Th22 cytokines). That is currently considered the "outside-in theory" (Silverberg and Silverberg 2015; Sullivan and Silverberg 2017).

On the other hand, supporters of the "inside-out theory" suggest that the immune system abnormalities in Th1/Th2 activity are the prime driver of AD. The activation of keratinocytes by environmental factors, for example, induces the release of thymic stromal lymphopoietin (TSLP). TSLP in turn activates dendritic cells, drives Th2 polarization, and enhances B cell differentiation and proliferation (Oyoshi et al. 2010). Th2 cytokines such as IL-4 and IL-13 promote the production of IgE by B cells, Th17, and Th22 and, consequently, the release of corresponding cytokines (Sullivan and Silverberg 2017). Th2 cytokines are known as STAT3 activators which induce FLG downregulation (Amano et al. 2005). Thus, elevated Th2 cytokines will contribute to the skin barrier breakdown.

ProFLG is a precursor of FLG, and FLG contributes to the formation of skin barrier. Recently, it has been suggested that products or drugs that could enhance FLG production would be of help in the management of AD (Otsuka et al. 2014; Choi et al. 2017); and sacran can be considered a natural skin barrier enhancer that could be useful in the treatment of skin disorders associated with skin barrier defect.

On the other hand, TNF-α, which is a key cytokine involved in the development of inflammatory diseases (AD included), is reported to induce TSLP expression in epidermal keratinocytes and to downregulate FLG production (Kim et al. 2011; Mizuno et al. 2015), thus contributing to the dysfunction of the skin barrier in AD patients. Given the anti-TNF-α effect of sacran, as shown in AD mouse models, it might be said that sacran not only ameliorates FLG production but also concomitantly prevents its downregulation. This double beneficial effect of sacran makes it a unique natural compound for skin health.

Sacran can penetrate the skin to reduce inflammation. We previously demonstrated in an experiment that sacran could be visualized in the rat paw skin after subcutaneous injection of λ-carrageenan solution (Fig. 8.12). Therefore in light of the foregoing, the anti-allergic effects of sacran could mainly be attributable to

(Hengge et al. 2006) its FLG production upregulation which enhances skin barrier function and accelerates skin barrier recovery (skin repair) and (Schoepe et al. 2006) its anti-TNF-α and anti-COX-2 activities, leading to the downregulation of the production of AD-triggering cytokines (Fig. 8.11). Nonetheless, extensive

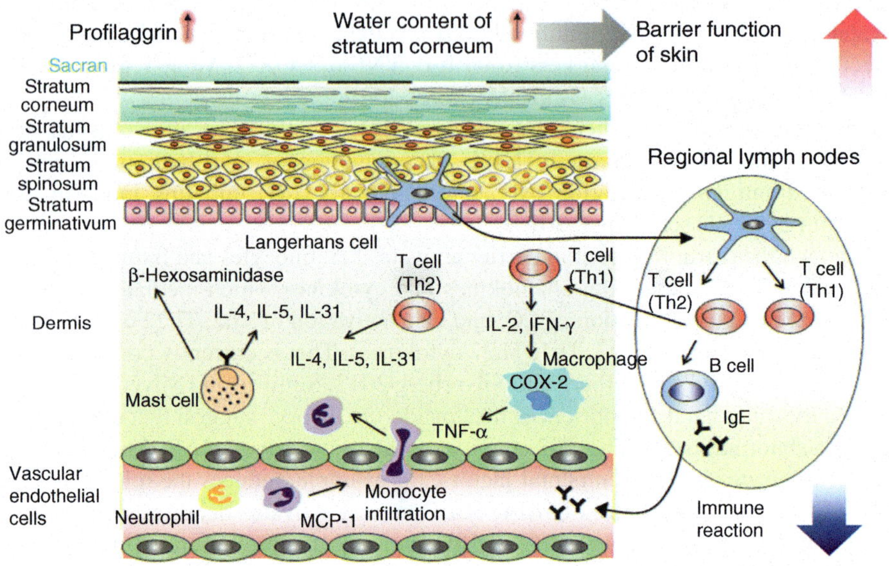

Fig. 8.11 Proposed anti-allergic mechanism of sacran. (Image developed by authors, Kumamoto University Graduate School of Pharm. Sciences, Japan)

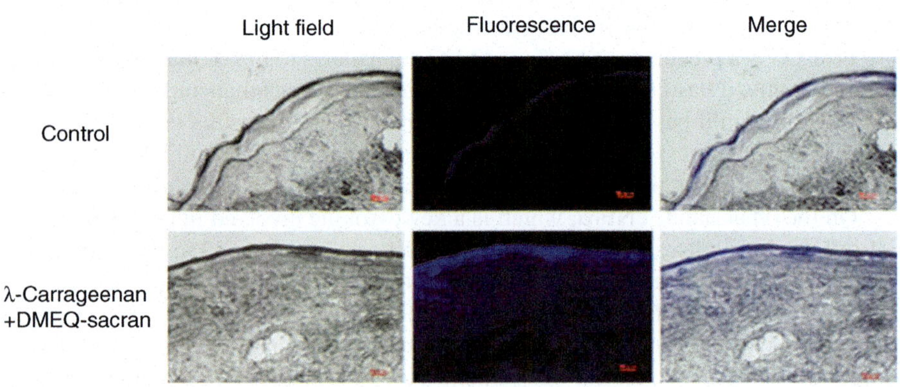

Fig. 8.12 Photographs of tissue slices of rat paw after treatment of DMEQ-labeled, sacran-labeled sacran solution (0.05% (w/v)) that was administered every 1 h after subcutaneous injection of λ-carrageenan solution to a rat paw. After 3 h, resected segments were observed with a fluorescent microscope (©The Pharmaceutical Society of Japan; with courtesy of Biological and Pharmaceutical Bulletin Editors). The figure shows that sacran can penetrate the stratum corneum of the skin, and that is particularly obvious for damaged skin by exogenous environmental factors including allergens and irritant substances

research is needed that will possibly determine receptors involved in the anti-inflammatory activity of sacran. Taken together, our findings suggest that sacran has a potential to serve as alternative natural anti-allergic adjuvant and therapeutic agent.

References

Amano W, Nakajima S, Kunugi H, et al. The Janus kinase inhibitor JTE-052 improves skin barrier function through suppressing signal transducer and activator of transcription 3 signaling. J Allergy Clin Immunol. 2005;136:667–77, e667.

Ananthi S, Raghavendran HR, Sunil AG, et al. In vitro antioxidant and in vivo anti-inflammatory potential of crude polysaccharide from Turbinaria ornata (Marine Brown Alga). Food Chem Toxicol. 2010;48:187–92.

Averbeck M, Gebhardt CA, Voight S, et al. Differential regulation of hyaluronan metabolism in the epidermal and dermal compartments of human skin by UVB irradiation. J Invest Dermatol. 2007;127:687–97.

Bernfield M, Gotte M, Park PW, et al. Functions of cell surface heparan sulfate proteoglycans. Annu Rev Biochem. 1999;68:729–77.

Choi HK, Cho YH, Lee EO, et al. Phytosphingosine enhances moisture level in human skin barrier through stimulation of the filaggrin biosynthesis and degradation leading to NMF formation. Arch Dermatol Res. 2017;309(10):795–803.

Fukushima S, Motoyama K, Tanida Y, et al. Clinical evaluation of novel natural polysaccharides Sacran as a skincare material for atopic dermatitis patients. J Cosmet Dermatological Sci Appl. 2016;6:9–18.

Gu H, Huang L, Wong YP, Burd A. HA modulation of epidermal morphogenesis in an organotypic keratinocyte-fibroblast co-culture model. Exp Dermatol. 2010;19:e336–9.

Hanifin JM. Evolving concepts of pathogenesis in atopic dermatitis and other eczemas. J Invest Dermatol. 2009;129:320–2.

Hengge UR, Ruzicka T, Schwartz RA, Cork MJ. Adverse effects of topical glucocorticosteroids. J Am Acad Dermatol. 2006;54:1–15; quiz 16-18.

Homey B, Steinhoff M, Ruzicka T, Leung DY. Cytokines and chemokines orchestrate atopic skin inflammation. J Allergy Clin Immunol. 2006;118:178–89.

Jin H, He R, Oyoshi M, Geha RS. Animal models of atopic dermatitis. J Invest Dermatol. 2009;129:31–40.

Kawashima H, Atarashi K, Hirose M, et al. Oversulfated chondroitin/dermatan sulfates containing GlcAb1/IdoAa1-3GalNAc(4,6-O-disulfate) interact with L- and P-selectin and chemokines. J Biol Chem. 2002;277:12921–30.

Kim BE, Howell MD, Guttman-Yassky E, et al. TNF-α downregulates filaggrin and loricrin through c-Jun N-terminal kinase: role for TNF-α antagonists to improve skin barrier. J Invest Dermatol. 2011;131(6):1272–9.

Kuschert GS, Coulin F, Power CA, et al. Glycosaminoglycans interact selectively with chemokines and modulate receptor binding and cellular responses. Biochemistry. 1999;38:12959–68.

Mizuno K, Morizane S, Takiguchi T, et al. Dexamethasone but not tacrolimus suppresses TNF-α-induced thymic stromal lymphopoietin expression in lesional keratinocytes of atopic dermatitis. Dermatol Sci. 2015;80(1):45–53.

Ngatu NR, Okajima MK, Yokogawa M, et al. Anti-inflammatory effects of sacran, a novel polysaccharide from Aphanothece sacrum, on 2,4,6-trinitrochlorobenzene-induced allergic dermatitis in vivo. Ann Allergy Asthma Immunol. 2012;108:117–22.

Ngatu NR, Hirota R, Okajima MK, et al. Sacran, a skin barrier enhancer, improves atopic and contact eczema: case repot. Ann Phytomed. 2015;4(1):111–3.

Ngatu NR, Tanaka M, Okajima MK, et al. Anti-allergic effects and immunomodulatory activity of sacran, a bioactive compound from river alga aphanothece sacrum. Evid Based Med Public Health. 2016;e1438:2.

Okajima MK, Bamba T, Kaneso Y, et al. Supergiant ampholytic sugar chains with imbalanced charge ratio form saline ultra-absorbent hydrogels. Macromolecules. 2008;41:4061–4.

Okajima MK, Kaneko D, Mitsumata T, et al. Cyanobacteria that produce megamolecules with efficient self-orientations. Macromolecules. 2009a;42:3057–62.

Okajima MK, Miyazato S, Kaneko T. Cyanobacterial megamolecule sacran efficiently forms LC gels with very heavy metal ions. Langmuir. 2009b;25:8526–31.

Okajima MK, Higashi T, Asakawa R, et al. Gelation behavior by the lanthanoid adsorption of the cyanobacterial extracellular polysaccharide. Biomacromolecules. 2010a;11:3172–7.

Okajima MK, Nakamura M, Mitsumata T, Kaneko T. Cyanobacterial polysaccharide gels with efficient rare-earth-metal sorption. Biomacromolecules. 2010b;11:1773–8.

Otsuka A, Doi H, Egawa G, et al. Possible new therapeutic strategy to regulate atopic dermatitis through upregulation of filaggrin expression. J Allergy Clin Immunol. 2014;133(1):139–46.

Oyoshi MK, Larson RP, Ziegler SF, et al. Mechanical injury polarizes skin dendritic cells to elicit a T(H)2 response by inducing cutaneous thymic stromal lymphopoietin expression. J Allergy Clin Immunol. 2010;126:976–84, 984.e1-5.

Parish CR. The role of heparan sulphate in inflammation. Nat Rev Immunol. 2006;6:633–43.

Park HY, et al. Anti-inflammatory effects of fucoidan through inhibition of NF-kappaB, MAPK and Akt activation in lipopolysaccharide-induced BV2 microglia cells. Food Chem Toxicol. 2011;49:1745–52.

Salmivirta M, Lidholt K, Lindahl U. Heparan sulfate: a piece of information. FASEB J. 1996;10:1270–9.

Schoepe S, Schacke H, May E, Asadullah K. Glucocorticoid therapy-induced skin atrophy. Exp Dermatol. 2006;15:406–20.

Seldin DC, Adelman S, Austen KF, et al. Homology of the rat basophilic leukemia cell and the rat mucosal mast cell. Proc Natl Acad Sci U S A. 1985;82:3871–5.

Silverberg NB, Silverberg JI. Inside out or outside in: does atopic dermatitis disrupt barrier function or does disruption of barrier function trigger atopic dermatitis? Cutis. 2015;96(6):359–61.

Sullivan M, Silverberg NB. Current and emerging concepts in atopic dermatitis pathogenesis. Clin Dermatol. 2017;35(4):349–53.

Taylor KR, Gallo RL. Glycosaminoglycans and their proteoglycans:host-associated molecular patterns for initiation and modulation of inflammation. FASEB J. 2006;20:9–22.

Visscher MO, Adam R, Brink S, et al. Newborn infant skin: physiology, development, and care. Clin Dermatol. 2015;33:271–80.

Volpi N. Therapeutic applications of glycosaminoglycans. Curr Med Chem. 2006;13:1799–810.

Yamada S, Sugahara K. Potential therapeutic application of chondroitin sulfate/dermatan sulfate. Curr Drug Discov Technol. 2008;5:289–301.

Yamashita H, Tasaki D, Makino T, et al. The role of IgE and repeated challenge in the induction of persistent increases in scratching behavior in a mouse model of allergic dermatitis. Eur J Pharmacol. 2009;605:153–7.

Yanase Y, Hiragun T, Uchida K, et al. Peritoneal injection of fucoidan suppresses the increase of plasma IgE induced by OVA-sensitization. Biochem Biophys Res Commun. 2009;387:435–9.

Chapter 9
Clinical Anti-Allergic Effects of African *Vernonia amygdalina* Leaf Extracts

Nlandu Roger Ngatu

Abstract *Vernonia amygdalina* Del. (VA) is an edible plant belonging to the Asteraceae family, genus *Vernonia*. This review mainly provides information about its effects on allergic skin disorders, namely, atopic and contact dermatitis. Leaf extracts of African *V. amygdalina* leaf contain several bioactive compounds, mainly flavonoids (luteolin, luteolin-7-O-glucuronide, luteolin 7-O-glucoside) and sesquiterpenes (*vernodalin*, *vernodalol*). It also contains a number of lipid and carbohydrates mainly threitol, inositol, hexadecanoic acid, and octadecanoic acid. After a personal experience on beneficial anti-inflammatory and anti-itch effects on skin disorders, we first conducted experimental studies using a mouse model of hapten-induced atopic dermatitis-like disease to evaluate the anti-itch and anti-allergic effects of VA leaf extracts. Later on, we conducted a preliminary comparative clinical trial in patients with atopic dermatitis (AD). In the prophylactic and curative studies in a mouse model of AD, *V. amygdalina* extracts (Vamex) displayed a better anti-itch effect than the steroid preparation (*hydrocortisone*), whereas it was as effective as *hydrocortisone* in regard to AD-like symptoms in mice. On the other hand, in a comparative preliminary clinical trial in African AD and CD patients, Vamex significantly reduced eczema area and severity index (EASI) and total serum immunoglobulin E (IgE) level as compared with Vaseline and was as effective as topical dexamethasone after a 2-week treatment period. Furthermore, our case reports on patients with complicated chronic and recalcitrant eczematous skin disorders also showed the beneficial effects of African *V. amygdalina* leaf-derived biomaterial on eczema, suggesting its potent anti-inflammatory and anti-allergic properties.

Keywords Atopic dermatitis · Contact dermatitis · Pruritus · *Vernonia amygdalina*

N. R. Ngatu, M.D., Ph.D. (✉)
Graduate School of Medicine, International University of Health and Welfare (IUHW), Chiba, Japan

Graduate School of Public Health, International University of Health and Welfare (IUHW), Tokyo, Japan

N. R. Ngatu, M. Ikeda (eds.), *Occupational and Environmental Skin Disorders*,
https://doi.org/10.1007/978-981-10-8758-5_9

Abbreviations

AD	Atopic dermatitis
CD	Contact dermatitis
EASI	Eczema area and severity index
ERK	Extracellular signal-regulated kinases
ESR	Erythrocyte sedimentation rate
GC-MS	Gas chromatography-mass spectroscopy
IgE	Immunoglobulin E
MAPK	Mitogen-activated protein kinases

9.1 Background

9.1.1 Epidemiological Profile of Atopic Dermatitis

Atopic dermatitis (AD) and contact dermatitis or contact eczema are prevalent skin diseases worldwide. AD often begins in infancy, and 45, 60, and 85% of children are thought to present with clinical AD symptoms by 6 months, 1 year, and 5 years of age, respectively (Bieber 2010). In children, AD prevalence has been increasing in children population, reaching 10–20%; and disease treatment consists mainly on the control of inflammation, the reduction of pruritus, and skin care (Lee et al. 2006; Kawakami et al. 2007; Bieber 2010; Ngatu et al. 2012). Although the prevalence of AD in Congolese children is not known, a screening conducted by Nyembue et al. (2012) by skin prick test (SPT) showed that allergen-sensitization rate in 423 children with rhinitis from Kinshasa, Democratic Republic of Congo (DRC), was 40.9% for polysensitization, 68.5% for *Dermatophagoides pteronyssinus*, and 36.2% for cockroach. This finding suggests that atopic status might be prevalent in Congolese children population.

9.1.2 Biological Properties and Chemical Composition of **Vernonia amygdalina** *Leaf*

Vernonia amygdalina Del. (Fig. 9.1) is an edible plant bot for humans and animals (mainly primates) in Africa, belonging to the Asteraceae family, genus *Vernonia*, which comprises more than 1000 species. The plant grows in the tropical Africa. Its leaf extracts (Vamex) contains several bioactive compounds, mainly flavonoids (luteolin, luteolin-7-O-glucuronide, luteolin 7-O-glucoside) and sesquiterpenes (*vernodalin*, *vernodalol*, *vernolepin*, *vernomygdin*, and *vernolides*) (Ijeh and CECC 2011). We also previously reported that Vamex contains lipid and carbohydrates, namely, threitol, inositol, hexadecanoic acid, and octadecanoic acid (Fig. 9.2)

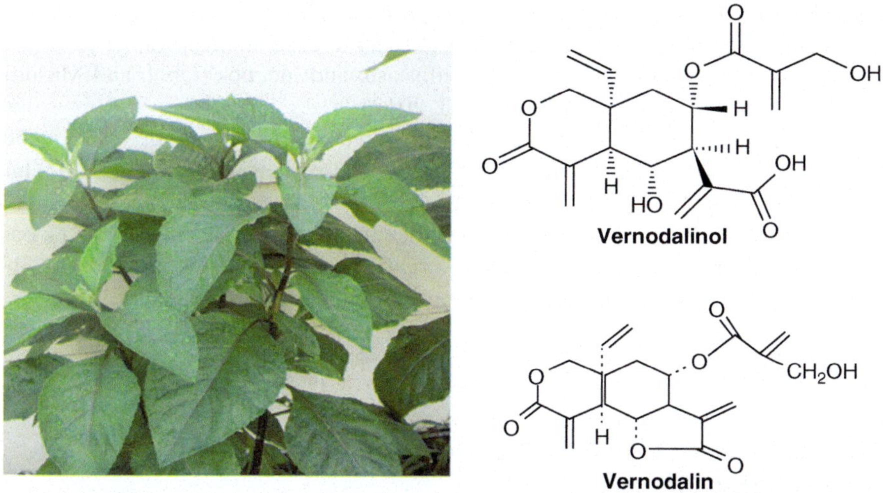

Fig. 9.1 Image of *Vernonia amygdalina* Del. and chemical structures of VA-derived bioactive anti-inflammatory sesquiterpene lactones, vernodalin and vernodalol (Luo et al. 2011; Ngatu et al. 2014a, b)

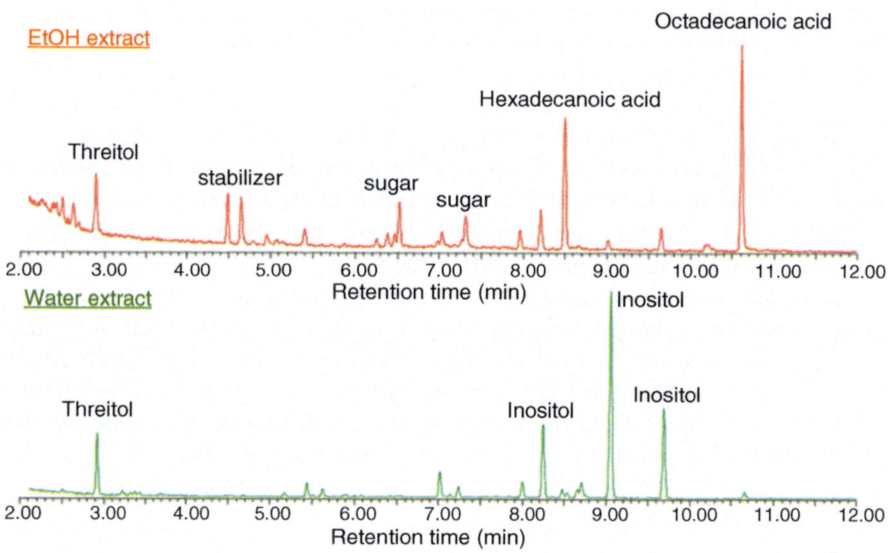

Fig. 9.2 GC-MS chromatogram of *Vernonia amygdalina* leaf ethanolic and water extracts Gas chromatography-mass spectroscopy (GC-MS) was performed to determine lipid and carbohydrate compounds in aqueous (Vamex1) and ethanolic (Vamex2) extracts of *Vernonia amygdalina* leaf at Kaneko Laboratory, ©Japan Advanced Institute of Science and Technology (JAIST).

(Ngatu et al. 2014a). In African ethnomedicine, the plant is used for wound healing and to treat a number of diseases such as gastrointestinal and respiratory disorders, malaria, diabetes, helminthiasis, kidney disease, and hiccups (Oboh and Masodje 2009; Olorunfemi et al. 2012; Ngatu et al. 2012).

Furthermore, a number of studies have shown that the ethanolic and aqueous *Vernonia amygdalina* leaf extracts have shown antioxidant (Erasto et al. 2007) and anticancer (Ezegbivie et al. 2004; Wong et al. 2013a) activities. These bioactive properties of *V. amygdalina* extracts have been attributed to its MAPK/ERK, caspase, and p53 pathway inhibitory effects (Oyugi et al. 2009; Wong et al. 2013b). However, there has been no scientific report on the beneficial effects of *V. amygdalina* on skin diseases.

9.2 Effects of African *Vernonia amygdalina* Leaf Extracts on Skin Allergy

9.2.1 Experimental Prophylactic and Curative Anti-Allergic Effects of Vernonia amygdalina *Leaf Extracts in Mouse Model of Atopic Dermatitis-Like Disease*

We recently published the first reports on the beneficial effects of Vamex on skin inflammatory diseases. In the prophylactic study on a mouse model of AD, *V. amygdalina* extracts (Vamex) displayed a good anti-itch effect (marked reduction of the number of scratching behaviors) (Fig. 9.3). In the curative protocol of the study, Vamex1 and Vamex2 were as effective as the steroid preparation (*hydrocortisone*) used in these experiments in alleviating AD-like skin lesions in mice (not shown). Both the water (Vamex1) and alcoholic (Vamex2) extracts of *V. amygdalina* leaf were equally effective (Ngatu et al. 2012, 2014b).

During the treatment period, controlled mice group had still a high average number of scratching behaviors, whereas they were significantly reduced in Vamex1, Vamex2, and hydrocortisone-treated mice groups ($p < 0.01$) (Ngatu et al. 2014a). The number of scratching behaviors in Vamex-treated groups was similar to that of normal mice group (not shown), and no significant difference was observed when comparing Vamex groups.

9.2.2 Clinical Anti-Itch and Anti-Allergic Effects of Vernonia Amygdalina *Leaf Extracts in Patients with Either Atopic or Allergic Contact Dermatitis (*N *= 25)*

In this preliminary comparative clinical trial, 25 patients with mild to moderate eczematous skin diseases (atopic dermatitis) were divided into 4 treatment groups of 5–7 patients (age range: 5–17 years). Within 1–2 weeks of topical treatment with

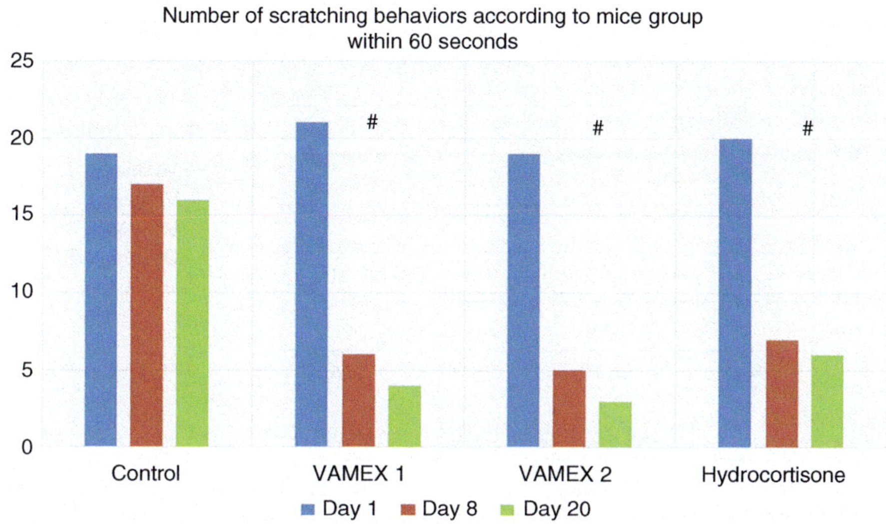

Fig. 9.3 Anti-itch effect of *Vernonia amygdalina* leaf extracts in the preventive protocol of a study on hapten-induced mouse model of atopic dermatitis-like disease. The figure shows reduced number of scratching behaviors in Vamex1 and Vamex2 mice groups compared to the untreated controlled mice group ($p < 0.01$). Similarly, hydrocortisone mice group also had reduced number of scratching behaviors (vs. control; $p < 0.01$). The number of scratching behaviors in Vamex groups was similar to that of normal group. On the other hand, though Vamex groups had lower scratching behavior counts than hydrocortisone-treated groups, no significant difference was observed when comparing the two groups

the water extracts (Vamex1), ethanolic extracts (Vamex2) of *V. amygdalina* leaf, or dexamethasone, pruritus was relieved in all patients (Fig. 9.4), and most of them had their skin condition alleviated by week 3 of treatment (Fig. 9.4b). In addition, none of the patients from Vamex and dexamethasone groups reported an adverse effect related to the treatment (Ngatu et al. 2014a). Furthermore, during the same study period, we also treated two patients (not included in the main study) with severe, chronic, and recalcitrant eczematous skin disorders with the use of topical Vamex. These cases are described below.

According to her mother, after a first visit at a local health center where a doctor told her parents that their daughter was suffering from psoriasis, she was treated using *betamethasone*-based product for months; however, skin lesions got progressively severe and recalcitrant. Then, her parents consulted a local healer who applied a plant-based herbal product for several months, which caused contact eczema and has contributed to the spread and worsening of skin lesions. She also developed scabies and tinea capitis later on. At the admission, she presented with disseminated scaly and dyschromic lesions, lichenification, and oozing on her back and upper and lower limbs. Tinea capitis lesions were visible on her head and neck (Fig. 9.5).

She was treated with topical 10% Vamex2 solution twice daily for eczematous and scabies lesions. For *tinea capitis* lesions, 2% miconazole was topically applied twice a day. Three weeks after the start of treatment, a marked amelioration of

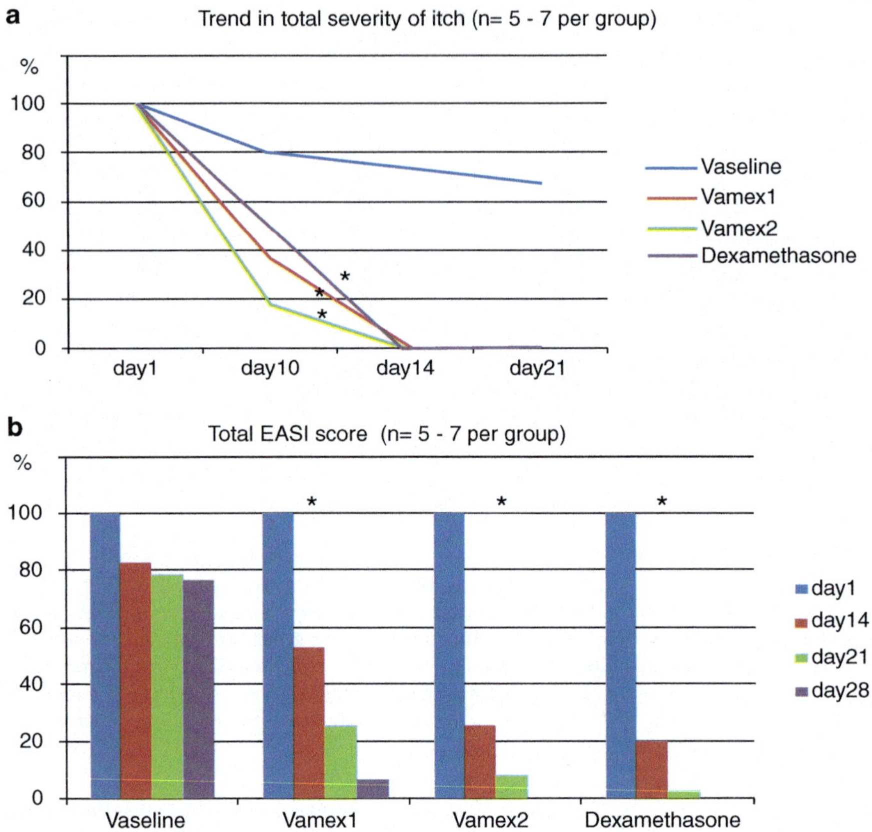

Fig. 9.4 (**a**, **b**) Total itch (**a**) and disease severity score (%) (**b**) according to treatment group ($N = 25$). The figure shows a complete relief of itch in patients treated with the alcoholic (Vamex2) and water (Vamex1) extracts of *Vernonia amygdalina* leaf, as well as dexamethasone, as compared with Vaseline. No significant difference was observed when comparing the anti-itch effects of Vamex1, Vamex2, and dexamethasone. In addition, Vamex1, Vamex2, and dexamethasone markedly reduced the eczema area and severity index (EASI) score as compared with Vaseline in allergic dermatitis patients with mild to moderate atopic dermatitis, and no significant difference was noted between Vamex and dexamethasone-treated groups (Ngatu et al. 2014b)

eczema area and severity index (EASI) score was observed, with a concomitant improvement of dermatological life quality index (DLQI) and a reduction of total serum immunoglobulin E (IgE) level and erythrocyte sedimentation rate (ESR) (Fig. 9.6) (Ngatu et al. 2014b).

The second patient was a 17-year-old albino boy from a village in Kongo Central (Bas-Congo) who presented with a chronic and recalcitrant photodermatitis. He reported that he was treated with topical betamethasone (most used remedy for skin diseases in this rural area) without any improvement. He had itchy skin rash, scratch markings, edema, and lichenified lesions on his neck and back. He was treated with

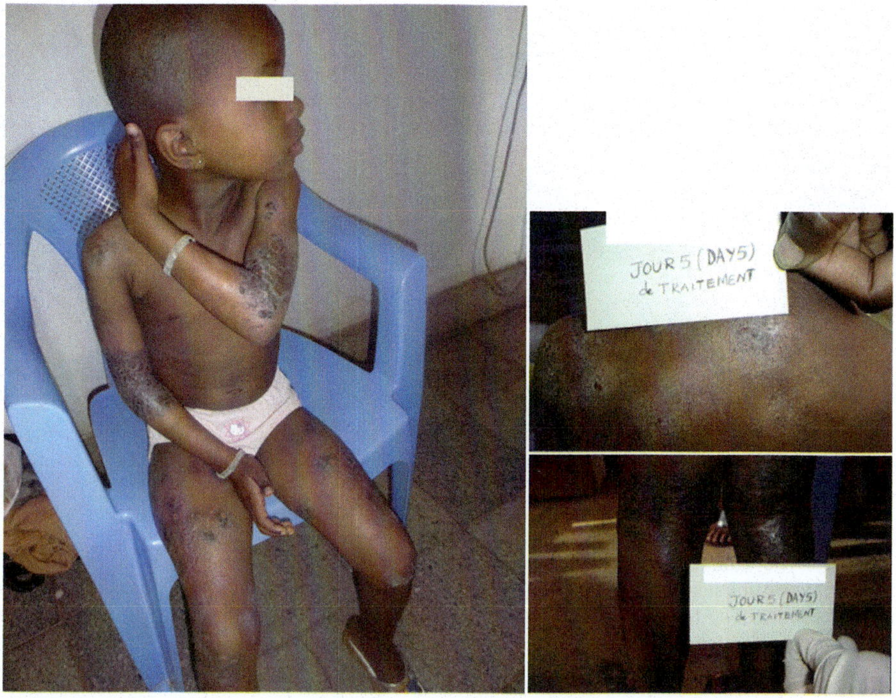

Fig. 9.5 Case of a 5-year-old Congolese girl with severe, chronic, and recalcitrant atopic dermatitis complicated with contact dermatitis and also scabies and tinea capitis (here are photos taken during the first week of Vamex treatment) (Ngatu et al. 2014b). The figure shows photos of body parts of a 5-year-old Congolese girl from Kongo Central province (formerly Bas-Congo province) whose parent consulted our "mobile clinic team" in rural Kongo Central in 2010. The girl has developed atopic dermatitis at age 1. Later on, it was complicated with contact eczema probably caused by the use of plant-based product from a local healer. She had difficulty to walk and could hardly play with friends

the use of topical 10% Vamex2. After a 3-week treatment period, his skin status improved considerably (Fig. 9.7) (Ngatu et al. 2012).

The case of chronic photodermatitis (Fig. 9.7) consisted of a 17-year-old boy from rural Kongo Central province in DRC who developed moderately itchy erythematous skin lesions with edema, lichenification, and excoriation about 3 months prior to his admission. Albinism is a congenital disorder characterized by a complete or partial absence of melanin, the pigment that provides normal color of the skin, hair, and eyes. The disorder is quite frequent in the sub-Saharan African region, and most albino individuals suffer from recurrent photodermatitis, sometimes skin cancer. The patient was treated at a local health center with topical betamethasone without any improvement. We treated him at the same health center with 10% Vamex2 which was administered topically twice a day for 4 weeks. His skin status improved after 3 weeks of treatment.

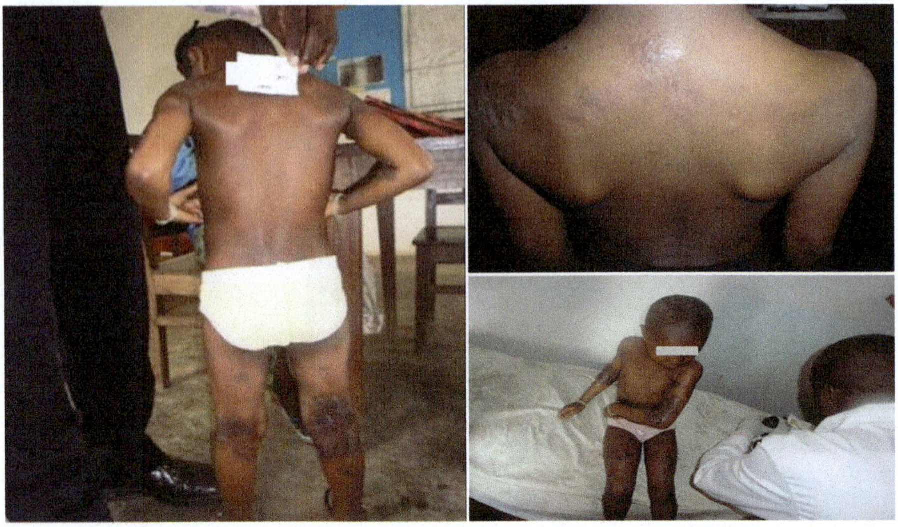

Fig. 9.6 The same 5-year-old Congolese patient after 3 weeks of treatment with topical 10% Vamex2 for trunk and upper and lower limbers skin lesions and topical 2% miconazole for tinea capitis lesions. The figure shows markedly reduced skin lesion severity mainly on the back and lower limbs. Her tinea capitis was cured (Ngatu et al. 2014a)

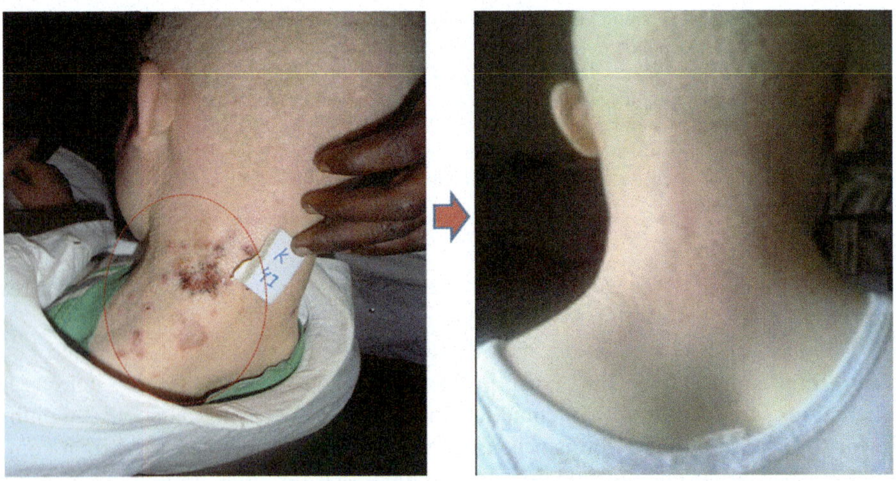

Fig. 9.7 Photodermatitis in a 17-year-old Congolese boy from rural Kongo Central province. This figure shows erythematous lesions on the neck with edema, lichenification, and excoriation at the admission (day1) and 3 weeks later, after topical treatment with 10% Vamex solution (Ngatu et al. 2012)

9.3 Discussion and Conclusion

In the present report, we highlighted the anti-itch, anti-inflammatory, and anti-allergic effects of biomaterials from the edible plant *Vernonia amygdalina* from DRC, which is used quite extensively in African ethnomedicine. Topical application of the plant extracts (Vamex) prevented the development of AD-like disease in hapten-challenged NC/Nga mice. In addition, Vamex alleviated skin lesions and suppressed pruritus in allergic NC/Nga mice as efficiently as *hydrocortisone* in the curative protocol of the experiment. Furthermore, topical Vamex relieved pruritus and suppressed skin lesions as efficiently as dexamethasone in patients with mild to moderate AD in a comparative clinical trial, as well as in two cases of chronic and recalcitrant dermatitis.

The discovery of natural products with anti-allergic properties similar to that of steroids and calcineurin inhibitors, without their adverse effects, has been the hope of many specialists in the field of allergy. Actually, not many plant-derived anti-allergic agents have been clinically effective in AD patients. A number of previous reports have suggested that biomaterials such as extracts and flavonoid fraction of chamomile applied topically have been effective in reducing croton oil-induced inflammation in rats (Dawid-Pac 2013). Additionally, a placebo-controlled randomized clinical trial on the efficacy of freeze-dried whey powder with spray-dried water extract of field dodder showed promising results in AD patients (Mehrbani et al. 2015). According to the authors, this natural product ameliorated AD skin lesions through improvement of the skin barrier function, reduced pruritus, and suppressed sleep disturbance in patients.

Currently, probiotics are attracting the interest of many allergologists given that they are providing clinical benefice to AD patients, according to recent investigations (Kalliomaki et al. 2001; Niccoli et al. 2014). A meta-analysis review of 25 randomized controlled studies on the management of AD with the use of probiotics showed improvement in disease severity score both in pediatric and adult patients (Kim et al. 2014). *Vernonia amygdalina* leaf contains terpenoid compounds that have been reported to exert anti-inflammatory and antitumor activity mainly through the inhibition of MAPK/ERK, caspase, and p53 pathways (Ezegbivie et al. 2004). In addition, its leaf extracts are known to possess antibacterial activity against *Staphylococcus aureus*, which colonizes the skin and is considered one of the factors that trigger AD. Our recent research (also reported in this work) has shown that topical application of *V. amygdalina*-derived biomaterial induced a marked increase expression of filaggrin, suggesting that it contains compounds that enhance the skin barrier. These facts suggest that *Vernonia amygdalina* could be a source of potential alternative natural anti-allergic agents.

Acknowledgments We thank Professor Narufumi Suganuma and Professor Hidetoshi Sano from Kochi University Medical School from the Department of Environmental Medicine and Department of Dermatology, respectively; we also thank Dr. Takao Saruta from Saruta Dermatological Clinic and Dr. Maki Yokogawa from Yokogawa Dermatological Clinic in Kochi prefecture, Japan, for their wonderful support during the implementation of our environmental allergic skin disorders research, which consisted of our PhD thesis theme.

Conflict of Interest: Findings from our *Vernonia amygdalina* and skin allergy research have been subject to patent application in 2010; an international and a national (Japan) patents were obtained in 2012 and 2015, respectively.

References

Bieber T. Atopic dermatitis. Ann Dermatol. 2010;22(2):125–37.

Dawid-Pac R. Medicinal plants used in treatment of inflammatory skin diseases. Postepy Dermatol Alergol. 2013;30(3):170–7.

Erasto P, Grierson DS, Afolayan AJ. Evaluation of antioxidant activity and the fatty acid profile of the leaves of Vernonia amygdalina growing in South Africa. Food Chem. 2007;104: 636–42.

Ezegbivie EB, Bryant JL, Walker A. A novel natural inhibitor of extracellular signal-regulated kinases and human breast cancer cell growth. Exp Biol. 2004;229:163–9.

Ijeh II, CECC E. Current perspectives on the medicinal potential of Vernonia. amygdalina. J Med Plants Res. 2011;5(7):1051–61.

Kalliomaki M, Salminen S, Arvilommi H, et al. Probiotics in primary prevention of atopic dermatitis: a randomized placebo-controlled trial. Lancet. 2001;357(9262):1076–9.

Kawakami Y, Yumoto K, Kawakami T. An improved mouse model of atopic dermatitis and suppression of skin lesions by an inhibitor of Tec family kinases. Allergol Int. 2007;56: 403–9.

Kim SO, Ah YM, Yu YM, et al. Effects of probiotics for the treatment of atopic dermatitis: a meta-analysis of randomized controlled trials. Ann Allergy Asthma Immunol. 2014;113(2): 217–26.

Lee SH, Kim SK, Han JB, et al. Inhibitory effects of Rumex japonicus Houtt on the development of atopic dermatitis-like skin lesions in NCNga mice. Br J Dermatol. 2006;155:33–83.

Luo X, Jiang Y, Frank R, et al. Isolation and structure determination of sesquiterpene lactone (vernodalinol) from Vernonia amygdalina extracts. Pharm Biol. 2011;49(5):464–70.

Mehrbani M, Choopani R, Fekri A, et al. The efficacy of whey associated with dodder extract on moderate-to-severe atopic dermatitis in adults: a randomized, double-blind, place-controlled clinical trial. J Ethnopharmacol. 2015;172:325–32.

Ngatu NR, Okajima MK, Yokogawa M, et al. Anti-allergic effects of Vernonia amygdalina leaf extracts on hapten-induced atopic dermatitis-like disease in mice. Allergol Int. 2012;61: 597–607.

Ngatu NR, Hirota R, Okajima MK, et al. Efficacy of leaf extracts of Vernonia amygdalina from Central Africa on atopic eczema. Ann Phytomed. 2014a;3(1):43–9.

Ngatu NR, Mukuamu M, Hirota R, et al. Severe, chronic and recalcitrant atopic dermatitis associated with tinea capitis: diagnostic approach and efficacy of topical Vernonia amygdalina Del. Extracts. Ann Phytomed. 2014b;3(1):103–6.

Niccoli AA, Artesi AL, Candio F, et al. Preliminary results on clinical effects of probiotic *Lactobacillus salivarius* LS01 in children affected by atopic dermatitis. J Clin Gastroenterol. 2014;48(1):S34–6.

Nyembue TD, Ntumba W, Omadjela LA, et al. Sensitization rate and clinical profile of Congolese patients with rhinitis. Allergy Rhinol. 2012;3(1):216–e24.

Oboh FOJ, Masodje HI. Nutritional and antimicrobial properties of Vernonia amygdalina leaves. Int J Biomed Health Sci. 2009;5(2):51–6.

Olorunfemi EA, Arnold IC, Chinenye I, et al. Effects of the leaf extracts of Vernonia amygdalina on the pharmacokinetics of dihydroartemisinin in rat. Pharmacologia. 2012;3(12):713–8.

Oyugi DA, Luo X, Lee KS, et al. Activity markers of the anti-breast carcinoma cell growth fractions of Vernonia amygdalina extracts. Exp Biol Med. 2009;234:410–7.

Wong GWK, Leung TF, Ko FWS. Changing prevalence of allergic diseases in the Asia-Pacific region. Allergy Asthma Immunol Res. 2013a;5(5):251–7.

Wong FC, Woo CC, Hsu A, et al. The anti-cancer activities of Vernonia amygdalina extracts in human breast cancer cell lines are mediated through caspase-dependent and p53-dependent pathways. PLoS One. 2013b;8(10):e78021.

Chapter 10
Experimental Anti-Allergic and Immunomodulatory Effects of *Vernonia amygdalina*-Derived Biomaterials, Vernodalin and Its Leaf Extracts

Ryoji Hirota and Nlandu Roger Ngatu

Abstract Atopic dermatitis (AD) is a chronic relapsing inflammatory skin disorder with a relatively high prevalence in children in developed countries. In this study, we (1) explored the immunomodulatory and (2) compared the anti-allergic effects of *Vernodalin* isolated from *Vernonia amygdalina* (VAM) leaf and VAM leaf extracts in NC/Nga mice. In the first experiment, AD-like disease was induced using 2,4,6-*trinitrochlorobenzene* (TNCB); the hapten was applied on mice rostral and ear's dorsal areas after disrupting skin barrier with the use of SDS solution. After AD induction, 36 NC/Nga mice that developed moderate to severe skin lesions were divided into 6 pretreatment groups of 6 animals: 1 μg/mL *Vernodalin*, 10 μg/mL *Vernodalin*, 100 μg/mL *Vernodalin*, 1,000 μg/mL VAM extracts, 1,000 μg/mL VAM extracts, and PBS-treated vehicle group. Skin samples were collected after 14 days of treatment; immunofluorescence and qRT-PCR assays were performed to determine changes in filaggrin (FLG) production and FLGmRNA and IL-33mRNA expressions, respectively. In the second experiment, 18 NC/Nga mice with *Dermatophagoides pteronyssinus* extract (DPE)-induced AD-like disease were divided into 3 treatment groups to test the curative effects of the experimental agents: 100 μg/mL *Vernodalin*, 10 μg/mL VAM extracts, and PBS-treated vehicle group as control.

Pretreatment with VAM extracts and Vernodalin caused an increase in FLGmRNA expression levels and a reduction of IL-33mRNA expression in mice (vs. control group). Furthermore, *Vernodalin* and VAM extracts significantly reduced the

R. Hirota, Ph.D. (✉)
Department of Nutrition, Matsumoto University, Nagano, Japan
e-mail: hirotar@kochi-u.ac.jp

N. R. Ngatu, M.D., Ph.D.
Graduate School of Medicine, International University of Health and Welfare (IUHW), Chiba, Japan

Graduate School of Public Health, International University of Health and Welfare (IUHW), Tokyo, Japan

N. R. Ngatu, M. Ikeda (eds.), *Occupational and Environmental Skin Disorders*,
https://doi.org/10.1007/978-981-10-8758-5_10

dermatitis score (vs. control) in regard to ear skin lesions. Findings from this study confirm the anti-allergic effects of VAM-derived bioactive compound, Vernodalin, and the plant extracts.

Keywords Atopic dermatitis · Hapten · NC/Nga mice · *Vernodalin* · *Vernonia amygdalina*

Abbreviations

ACD	Allergic contact dermatitis
AD	Atopic dermatitis
DPE	*Dermatophagoides pteronyssinus* extracts
FLG	Filaggrin
HPRT	Hypoxanthine phosphoribosyltransferase
IL	Interleukin
mRNA	Messenger ribonucleic acid
qRT-PCR	Quantitative real-time polymerase chain reaction
VAM	*Vernonia amygdalina*

10.1 Introduction

Allergic skin disorders such as atopic dermatitis (AD) and allergic contact dermatitis (ACD) are influenced by the imbalance between Th-1 and Th-2 cytokines production; they have recently been associated with an upregulation of IL-33 production (Yokozeki et al. 2003; Meephansan et al. 2012). IL-33, the most recently discovered member of the IL-1 family, is implicated in type 2 T-helper cell immune reactions and induces dendritic cells activation to external stimuli (Cayrol and Girard 2009; Meephansan et al. 2012), and its expression in the skin is reported to play an important role in the pathogenesis of allergic inflammation (Imai et al. 2013). On the other hand, a defect in the skin barrier which is caused by loss-of-function mutations in the gene responsible for filaggrin (FLG) production, a filament-aggregating protein encoded by the FLG gene, is reported to play a part (Smith et al. 2006; Brown and McLean 2012; Margolis et al. 2012), particularly in the pathogenesis of AD.

Vernonia amygdalina (VAM) is used in African ethnomedicine as a remedy for a number of conditions such as fever, malaria, diabetes, kidney disease, gastrointestinal disorders, kidney disorders, and hepatitis (Oboh 2009; Olorunfemi et al. 2012). Previous reports on the antitumor activity of *V. amygdalina* (VAM) leaf extracts, particularly on breast cancer, are said to be promising (Izevbigie et al. 2004). We previously reported the anti-allergic effects of VAM extracts (Ngatu et al. 2012). On the other hand, *Vernodalin*, a terpenoid compound isolated from VAM and other plant materials, is known to play a role in the anti-inflammatory activity of VAM extracts and is also reported to exert antitumor effects in vitro via caspase pathway (Looi et al. 2013). The present work evaluated the anti-allergic, as well as FLG and IL-33 production modulatory effects of *Vernodalin* isolated from *V. amygdalina* and VAM extracts in NC/Nga mice.

10.2 Materials and Methods

10.2.1 Animal Experiments

10.2.1.1 Protocol 1 of the Animal Experiment: Efficacy Comparison of Vernodalin and VAM Extracts on Dermatophagoides pteronyssinus Extract (DPE)-Induced Dermatitis in Mice

Thirty female NC/Nga mice (Charles River, Japan) aged 9 weeks were first sensitized with an ointment containing DPE, commercialized under the name of Biostir AD (Biostir, Kobe, Japan) as previously reported (Yamamoto et al. 2009; Yun et al. 2010). Briefly, mice were shaved to induce dermatitis on rostral area with the use of an electric clipper, and the remaining hair was depilated using hair removal cream. Skin barrier was disrupted with 150 mL 4% SDS solution before exposure to DPE. A week after the first exposure to the allergen (sensitization), they were challenged to DPE twice a week for 2 weeks to induce the dermatitis (Fig. 10.1). Eighteen mice with moderate to severe dermatitis were divided into three groups of six mice: 10 μg/mL VAM extracts, 100 g/ mL *vernodalin*, and phosphate-buffered solution (PBS)-treated control group.

The scoring of the severity of the dermatitis was evaluated as previously described (Yamamoto et al. 2009): each of the following skin lesions—erythema/hemorrhage, scarring/dryness, edema, and excoriation/erosion—was scored as 0 (none), 1 (mild), 2 (moderate), or 3 (severe); the sum of individual scores was equivalent to the overall

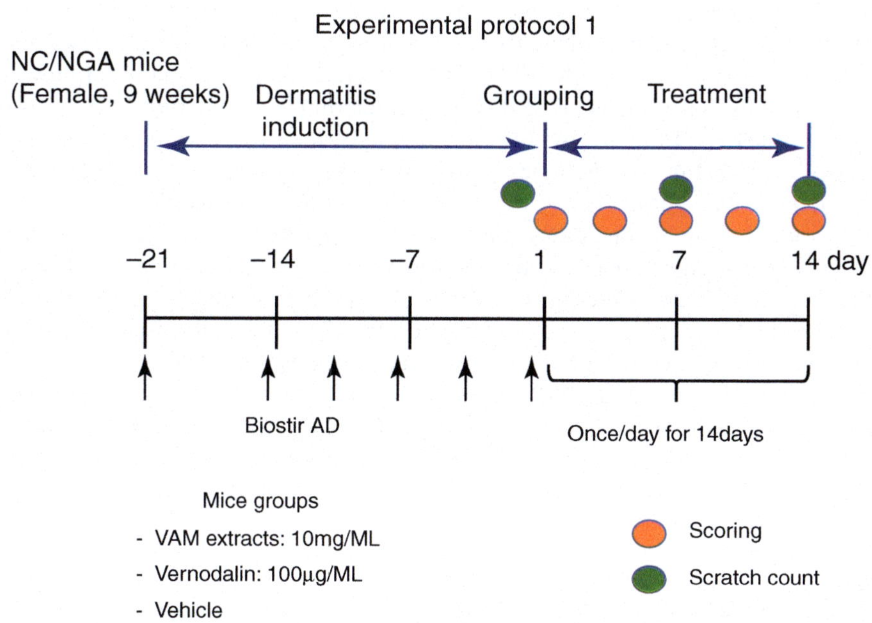

Fig. 10.1 Experimental protocol on the anti-inflammatory effects of Vernodalin and acetone extracts of Vernonia amygdalina leaf on Dermatophagoides pteronyssinus extract-induced dermatitis in mice

dermatitis score. The left ear skin samples to be used for histopathological examination were fixed in 10% formalin, embedded in paraffin. Mice were sectioned at 5 μm, and the specimens were stained with hematoxylin and eosin.

10.2.1.2 Protocol 2 of Vernodalin and Extracts of *Vernonia amygdalina* (VAM) on Ilaggrin (FLG) and IL-33 Production in Mice

(a) *Dermatitis Induction*

In this experiment, 40 female NC/Nga mice (Charles River, Japan), aged 9 weeks, have also been exposed to 2,4,6-*trinitrochlorobenzene* (TNCB) to induce dermatitis. However, prior to allergen exposure, a pretreatment (*Vernodalin*, VAM extracts, or PBS) was administered at the start of experiment and then continuously until completing 12 h.

Thirty-six NC/Nga mice that developed moderate to severe skin lesions were divided into six treatment groups of six animals: 100 μg/mL VAM extracts, 1,000 μg/mL VAM extracts, 1 μg/mL Vernodalin, 10 μg/mL Vernodalin, 100 μg/mL Vernodalin, and PBS-treated acetone (vehicle) group. The treatments were administered topically once a day for 2 weeks. Clinical evaluation was performed at days 1, 7, and 14 of the treatment period; the scoring of the dermatitis severity in mice was evaluated as described in protocol 1. All mice were sacrificed by anesthesia on day 14 of treatment period.

(b) *Quantitative Real-Time Polymerase Chain Reaction (qRT-PCR)*

Skin biopsies from allergen-exposed body areas were collected after 6 and 12 h on day 1 and also after 14 days for immunological assays. Quantitative real-time polymerase chain reaction (qRT-PCR) was performed using skin samples following the method by Nakajima et al. (2011) for the determination of expression levels of IL-33 mRNA and FLGmRNA (Fig. 10.2). Briefly, total RNA was extracted using TRIzol reagent (Life Technologies, Carlsbad, CA) according to the manufacturer's instructions; then purified RNA was reverse transcribed by SuperScript III reverse transcriptase (Life Technologies, Carlsbad, CA). Tenfold serial dilutions of templates were prepared in sterile water and were used as templates for qRT-PCR. These qRT-PCR experiments were carried out based on a Life technologies StepOnePlus™ real-time PCR system (Life Technologies, Carlsbad, CA) with the use of Assay-on-Demand gene expression products (Life Technologies, Carlsbad, CA) for IL-33 mRNA (00434203) and FLGmRNA according to the manufacturer's recommendations. The quantity of each transcript was analyzed using the StepOne™ Software V 2.1 (Life Technologies, Carlsbad, CA) and normalized to hypoxanthine phosphoribosyltransferase (HPRT) rRNA according to the ΔΔCt method.

10.2.2 Immunochemical Assay

The immunohistochemical staining for filaggrin was performed using the ABC Technique, as previously 7 described (Cheng et al. 2007). The paraffin-embedded tissue samples from mice were cut at 5 μm and placed on frosted microscope slides;

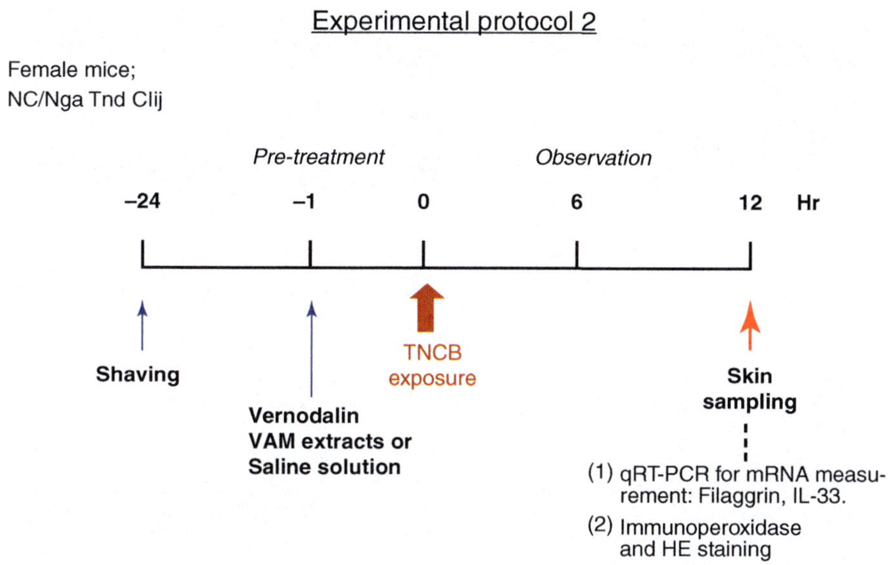

Fig. 10.2 Experimental protocol on the effects of Vernodalin and acetone extracts of Vernonia amygda lina leaf on FLGmRNA, TNF-α mRNA, IL-33mRNA, and immunoglobulin E (IgE) mRNA expression

later on, the slides were deparaffinized with the use of a series of xylene and ethanol washes and then stained using the VECTASTAIN Elite ABC Kit (Vector Laboratories, Burlingame, CA). The endogenous peroxidase was blocked by incubating the slides with 0.3% H_2O_2 for 10 min, and then tissue sections blockade was performed using normal serum for 15 min. The slides were then stained overnight with a polyclonal rabbit anti-mouse filaggrin antibody (Abcam, Cambridge, MA) at a 1:500 dilution. The biotinylated secondary antibody and NovaRED stain were added according to the manufacturer's protocol (Vector Laboratories, Burlingame, CA). The intensity of the immunostaining was graded with the use of microscopy on a scale from 0 to 5, with 0 indicating no staining and 5 the most intense staining (Fig. 10.3).

10.2.3 Ethical Consideration and Statistical Analyses

Both experiments were approved and performed in conformity with the ethical guidelines of the Kochi Medical School Animal Laboratory.

Data are expressed as mean ± SD, and for clinical score and biological markers, the statistical differences were assessed with the use of unpaired *t* test followed by Dunnett's test. All statistical analyses were performed with the use of Stata package version 10 (STATA Corp., TX, USA). The significance level of the difference between treatment groups was set at $p < 0.05$.

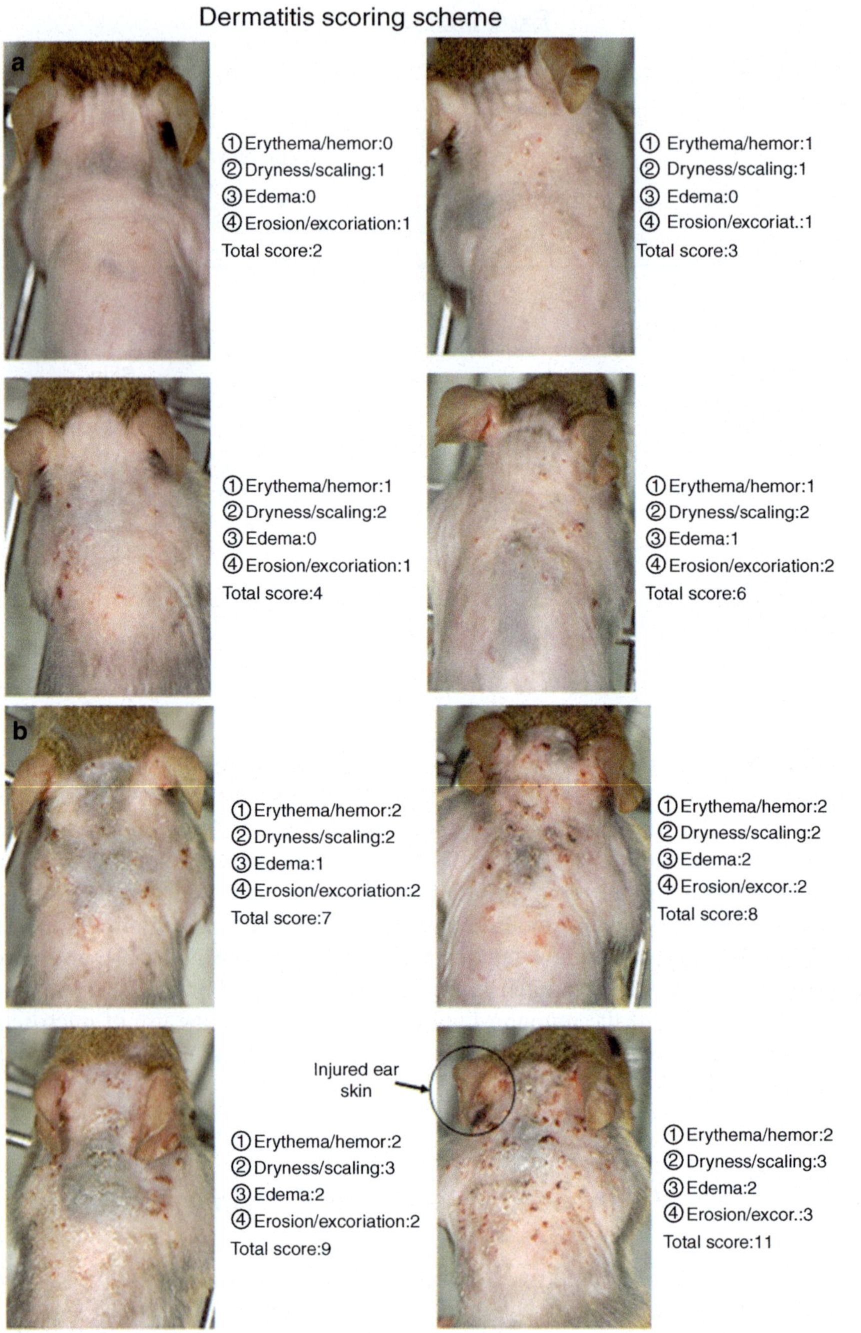

Fig. 10.3 (**a**, **b**) Images showing how to evaluate the severity of hapten-induced dermatitis in mice. In this figure, the severity of each of the skin lesions (erythema/hemorrhage, dryness/scaling, erosion/excoriation, edema) was first determined using a four-point scale (0–3), and then the sum of scores for all lesions made the total severity score for each mouse

10.3 Results

10.3.1 Severity of the Dermatitis and Effects of Topical Vernodalin and VAM in Allergic Mice

As mentioned in the methods section, the severity of the dermatitis was evaluated using of a "dermatitis scoring scheme" in each of the skin lesions (scaling/dryness, erythema/hemorrhage, edema, erosion/excoriation); for each skin lesion, four levels of severity were considered, 0 (absence), 1 (mild), 2 (moderate), and 3 (severe), separately for ears and the rostral area. The sum of individual scores was taken as the overall dermatitis score for ear or rostral area's skin lesions.

Topical application of 0.1 mg/mL Vernodalin and 10 mg/ml VAM significantly reduced the total severity score of ear skin lesions as compared with the vehicle ($p < 0.01$). When comparing Vernodalin and VAM extracts group, no statistically significant difference was found ($p > 0.05$) (Fig. 10.4a). On the other hand, in regard to rostral skin lesions, topical 0.1 mg/mL Vernodalin displayed a better anti-inflammatory effect with marked reduction of the total dermatitis severity score as compared with the vehicle ($p < 0.01$) and VAM extract ($p < 0.05$)-treated mice

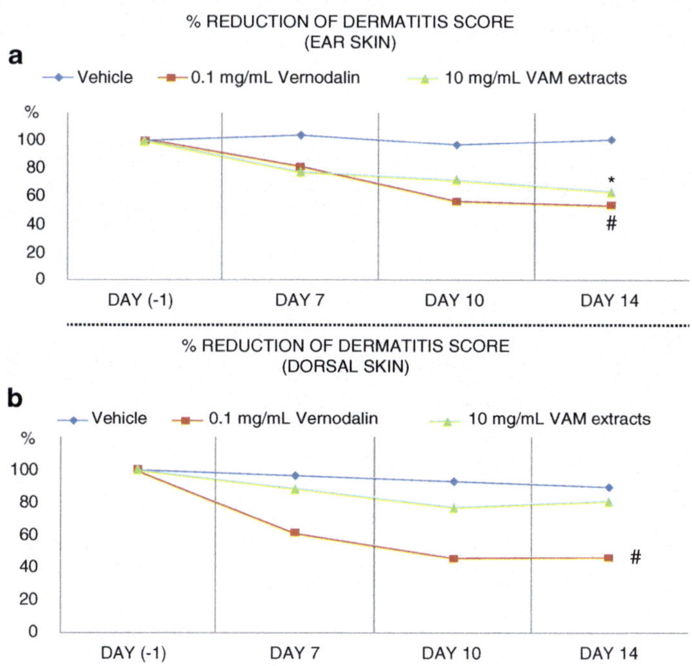

Fig. 10.4 (**a**, **b**) Effects of topical Vernodalin and VAM extracts on Dermatophagoides pteronyssinus extract-induced ear (**a**) and dorsal area (**b**) dermatitis skin lesions in NC/Nga mice. The figure shows markedly reduced dermatitis severity score in 0.1 mg/mL Vernodalin and 10 mg/mL VAM extracts' ear skin lesions, whereas, for rostral skin lesions, a significant decrease of dermatitis severity was observed only for 0.1 mg/mL Vernodalin ($p < 0.01$)

groups. In addition, though VAM extracts showed a relatively better effect within the first week of treatment, no statistically significant difference was noted when comparing VAM extracts and vehicle groups at the end of experiment (Fig. 10.4b). In addition, both Vernodalin and VAM extract-treated mice had reduced scratch count as compared to the vehicle group ($p < 0.05$) (not shown).

10.3.2 Effects of Topical Vernodalin and VAM Extracts on Filaggrin (FLG) Production (HE and Immunostaining) and FLGmRNA and IL-33 mRNA Expression in Mice

Filaggrin (FLG), one of important proteins of the *stratum corneum*, plays an important role in skin barrier function. For the restoration of a damaged skin barrier, a subsequent increase in filaggrin production is necessary. In this experiment, the HE stained mouse skin samples showed an intense cell infiltration and still severely injured skin, with destructed and hemorrhagic *stratum corneum*, in the control (TNCB) mice, whereas those processed were markedly reduced in mice treated with high concentration of Vernodalin (10 μg/mL and 100 μg/mL Vernodalin) and VAM extracts (100 μg/mL and 1,000 μg/mL VAM) (vs. control mice) (Fig. 10.5a–c). Similarly, the

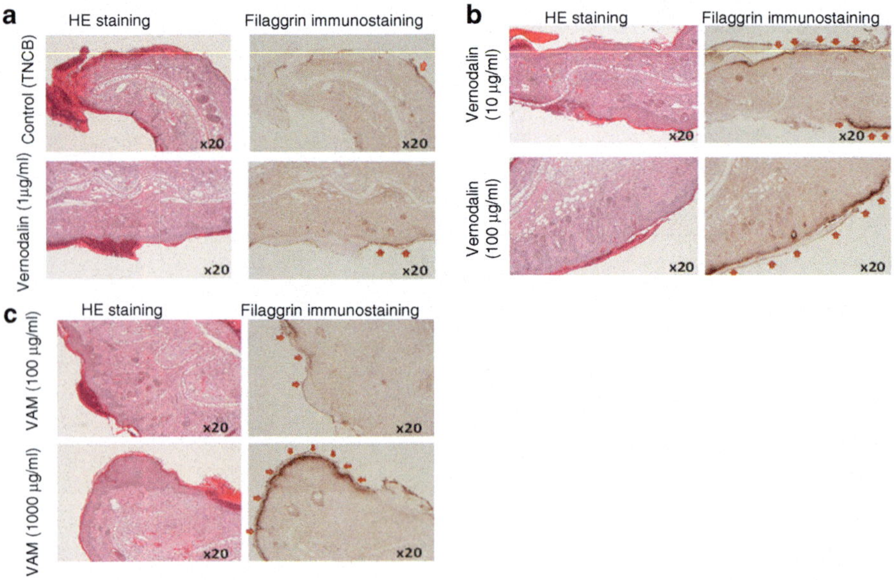

Fig. 10.5 (**a**–**c**) Filaggrin (FLG) production as visualized by immunostaining in Vernodalin and VAM mice. The figures show HE images with reduced inflammatory process in μg/mL Vernodalin (**b**) and. 1,000 μg/mL VAM extracts (**c**) in mice ear skin in the representative control mouse's ear; on the other hand, immunostaining images show enhanced FLG production in 100 μg/mL and 1,000 μg/mL VAM. (**c**) and 10 μg/mL and 100 μg/mL Vernodalin in mice (**b**)

immunoperoxidase staining of skin samples also showed an increased FLG expression in the skin of the corresponding Vernodalin and VAM mice (Fig. 10.5b, c).

Additionally, qRT-PCR analysis showed a markedly increased expression of FLGmRNA particularly in mice treated with high concentration of Vernodalin (100 μg/mL or 0.1 mg/mL Vernodalin) and VAM extracts (1,000 μg/mL or 1 mg/mL VAM extracts) as compared with respective lower concentration groups (Fig. 10.6a). This amelioration of FLG expression might be responsible of the advanced regeneration of the skin observed in 0.1 mg/mL (or 100 μg/mL) Vernodalin, 0.1 mg/mL (or 100 μg/mL) VAM extracts, and 1 mg/mL (or 1,000 μg/mL) VAM extract-treated mice, suggesting a progressive skin barrier repair activity. Furthermore, results of immunoperoxidase staining showed a noticeable decrease of IL-33mRNA expression level in all Vernodalin and VAM extract-pretreated mice groups as compared to the control group. Moreover no statistically significant difference was observed when comparing 0.1 mg/mL Vernodalin, 0.1 mg/mL VAM extracts, and 1 mg/mL VAM extracts mice groups.

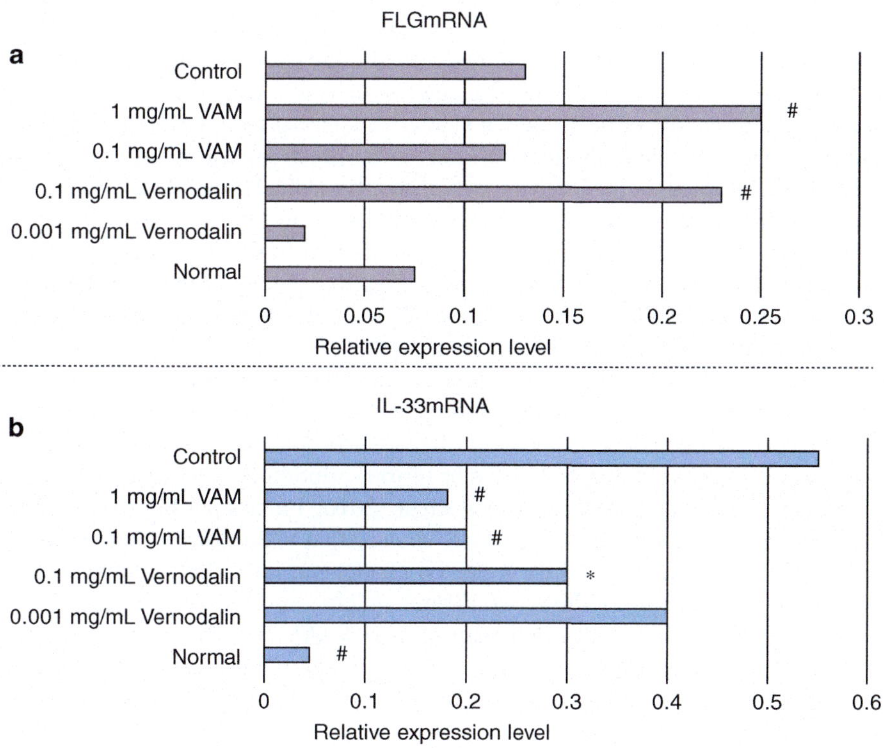

Fig. 10.6 (**a**, **b**). Filaggrin (FLG)-mRNA and IL-33mRNA expression levels as determined by qRT-PCR in. Vernodalin and VAM extract-treated mice. # p-value less than 0.01; *p-value less than 0.05; FLG, filaggrin; mRNA, messenger ribo nucleic acid; VAM, Vernonia amygdalina. Figure 10.5 (**a**, **b**) shows remarkable increase in FLGmRNA expression level in 1 mg/mL VAM extracts and 0.1 mg/mL Vernodalin mice group (vs. control group). On the other hand, regarding IL-33mRNA, its expression was markedly reduced in 0.1 mg/mL VAM extracts, 1 mg/mL VAM extracts, and 0.1 m/mL Vernodalin mice groups (vs. control (**a**, **b**))

10.4 Discussion and Conclusion

The present report consists of two experiments on allergen and hapten-induced AD-like disease that showed that topical treatment with Vernodalin and VAM extracts reduced dermatitis severity score in diseased mice, with Vernodalin displaying a better anti-allergic activity than VAM extracts. On the other hand, histological examination of skin samples from mice exposed to the hapten after pretreatment with VAM extracts and Vernodalin showed increased FLGmRNA and reduced IL-33mRNA expression levels.

We have previously demonstrated both in animal and clinical studies that VAM, whose main bioactive compound is *Vernodalin*, has anti-inflammatory and anti-itch effects on atopic and contact dermatitis. The new finding from the present work is that VAM and also Vernodalin induced an increase in FLGmRNA expression. This finding suggests that VAM has a good skin barrier repair activity. Considering its anti-inflammatory property and anti-bacterial activity mainly against gram+ (Okigbo and Mmeka 2008) that mostly colonize atopic skin, VAM could be an alternative natural anti-allergic candidate for the management of allergic skin disorders.

Steroids represent the first-line remedy for allergic skin disorders; however, their cautious utilization is recommended given the adverse effects they induce in some patients. And one of steroids' known side effects is that they may cause skin atrophy, which leads to the impairment of skin barrier function. Anti-allergic agents that display FLG upregulating activity are currently scarcely found. We previously reported that sacran, a new natural glycosaminoglycan-like compound from river alga *Aphanothece sacrum*, has anti-inflammatory and FLG upregulating properties (Ngatu et al. 2017). Other studies have suggested that emollients improved skin barrier recovery (Ghadially et al. 1992; Lodén 2003) and enhanced corticosteroid therapy in AD children (Szczepanowska et al. 2008).

IL-33 is a newly recognized cytokine of the IL-1 family, released by epithelial cells in various tissues, including keratinocytes and immune cells. It is reported to drive Th2 response in allergic and atopic diseases through the activation of signaling pathways signal transducer and activator of transcription 5, mitogen-activated protein kinase, NF-κB, and Akt (Ivanov et al. 2010; Funakoshi-Tago et al. 2011; Cevikbas and Steinhoff 2012). This study showed that VAM extracts and Vernodalin reduced IL-33mRNA expression in hapten-challenged mice. This finding supports the anti-allergic activity of those two natural agents.

This study is the first to demonstrate that VAM extracts, which have anti-inflammatory and anti-bacterial effects, and Vernodalin modulate FLGmRNA and IL-33mRNA expressions, suggesting their potential as alternative natural therapeutic anti-allergic agents.

References

Brown SJ, McLean WH. One remarkable molecule: filaggrin. J Invest Dermatol. 2012;132:751–62.
Cayrol C, Girard JP. The IL-1-like cytokine IL-33 is inactivated after maturation by caspase-1. Proc Natl Acad Sci. 2009;106:9021–6.

Cevikbas F, Steinhoff M. IL-33: a novel danger signal system in atopic dermatitis. J Invest Dermatol. 2012;132(5):1326–9.
Cheng YM, Wu MF, Wang J, et al. Human papillomavirus 16/18 E6 oncoprotein is expressed in lung cancer and related with p53 inactivation. Cancer Res. 2007;15:10686–93.
Funakoshi-Tago M, Tago K, Sato Y, et al. JAK2 is an important signal transducer in IL-33-induced NF-kappaB activation. Cell Signal. 2011;23:363–70.
Ghadially R, Halker-Sorensen L, Elias PM. Effects of petrolatum on stratum corneum structure and function. J Am Acad Dermatol. 1992;26(3):387–96.
Imai Y, Yasuda K, Sakaguchi Y, et al. Skin-specific expression of IL-33 activates group 2 innate lymphoid and elicits atopic dermatitis-like inflammation in mice. Proc Natl Acad Sci. 2013;110(34):13921–6.
Ivanov VN, Zhou H, Ghandhi SA, et al. Radiation-induced bystander signaling pathways in human fibroblasts: a role for interleukin-33 in the signal transmission. Cell Signal. 2010;22:1076–87.
Izevbigie EB, Bryant JL, Walker A. A novel natural inhibitor of extracellular signal-regulated kinases and human breast cancer cell growth. Exp Biol. 2004;229:163–9.
Lodén M. The skin barrier and use of moisturizers in atopic dermatitis. Clin Dermatol. 2003;21(2):145–57.
Looi CY, Arya A, Cheah FK, et al. Induction of apoptosis in human breast cancer cells via caspase pathway by Vernodalin isolated from Centratherum anthelminticum (L.) seeds. PLoS One. 2013;8(2):e56643.
Margolis DJ, Apter AJ, Gupta J, et al. The persistence of atopic dermatitis and Filaggrin mutations in a US longitudinal cohort. J Allergy Clin Immunol. 2012;130(4):912–7.
Meephansan J, Tsuda H, Komine M, Tominaga S, Ohtsuki M. Regulation of IL-33 expression by IFN-g and tumor necrosis factor-a in normal human keratinocytes. J Invest Dermatol. 2012;132:2593–600.
Nakajima K, Kanda T, Takaishi M, Shiga T, Miyoshi K, Nakajima H, et al. Distinct roles of IL-23 and IL-17 in the development of psoriasis-like lesions in a mouse model. J Immunol. 2011;186:448–4489.
Ngatu NR, Okajima MK, Yokogawa M, et al. Anti-allergic effects of Vernonia amygdalina leaf extracts in hapten-induced atopic dermatitis-like disease in mice. Allergol Int. 2012;61(4):597–607.
Ngatu NR, Motoyama K, Nishimura Y, et al. Anti-allergic and profilaggrin (proFLG)-mRNA expression modulatory effects of sacran. Int J Biol Macromol. 2017;105(Pt2):1532–8.
Oboh FOJ, Masodje HI. Nutritional and antimicrobial activities of Vernonia amygdalina leaves. Int J Biomed Health Sci. 2009;5(2):51–6.
Okigbo RN, Mmeka EC. Antimicrobial effects of three tropical plant extracts on Staphylococcus aureus, Escherichia coli and Candida albicans. Afr J Tradit Complement Altern Med. 2008;5(3):226–9.
Olorunfemi EA, Igboasoiyi A, Chinenye I, et al. Effects of leaf extracts of Vernonia amygdalina on the pharmacokinetics of dihydroartemisinin in rats. Pharmacologia. 2012;3(12):713–8.
Smith FJ, Irvine AD, Terron-Kwiatkowski A, et al. Loss-of-function mutations in the gene encoding Filaggrin cause ichthyosis vulgaris. Nat Genet. 2006;38(3):337–42.
Szczepanowska J, Reich A, Szepietowski JC. Emollients improve treatment results with topical corticosteroids in childhood atopic dermatitis: a randomized comparative study. Pediatr Allergy Immunol. 2008;19(7):614–8.
Yamamoto M, Haruna T, Ueda C, et al. Contribution of itch-associated scratch behavior to the development of skin lesions in dermatophagoides farina-induced dermatitis model in NC/Nga mice. Arch Dermatol Res. 2009;301:739–46.
Yokozeki H, Wu MH, Sumi K, et al. Th2 cytokines, IgE and mast cells play a crucial role in the induction of para-phenylenediamine-induced contact hypersensitivity in mice. Clin Exp Immunol. 2003;132:385–92.
Yun MY, Yang JH, Kim DK, et al. Therapeutic effects of Baicalein on atopic dermatitis-like skin lesions of NC/Nga mice induced by dermatophagoides pteronyssinus. Int Immunopharmacol. 2010;10(9):1142–8.

Part III
Fungal, Neglected Seasonal, Epidemic and Other Environmental Skin Disorders

Chapter 11
Common Environmental Dermatomycoses

Nlandu Roger Ngatu

Abstract Environmental fungal skin disorders (EFSD) or dermatomycoses have a worldwide distribution, with high prevalence in most developing countries. Causal agents include dermatophytes and opportunistic fungi (*Malassezia*, *Candida*, *Trichosporon*, *Rhodotorula*, *Cryptococcus* or *Aspergillus*, *Geotrichum*, *Alternaria*, etc.). Besides their specific risk factors, common superficial dermatomycoses share common group of associated factors, such as "environmental and geographical factors" (climate, humidity), "human factors" (population mobility, personal hygiene, abusive use of antifungal drugs), and "economic factor" (poverty), which determine their distribution in regions of the world. *Trichophyton interdigitale*, *T. tonsurans*, and *M. canis* are getting more frequent globally. High prevalence rate of *T. capitis* has been reported in African children: 50–54% in rural Ethiopia, 11.2% in rural Democratic Republic of the Congo (DRC), 7.4% in Egypt, and 7.1% in Tanzania, whereas rates of 3–8% have been found in the United States. The clinical diagnosis of *T. capitis* is made in the presence of dry scaling-like dandruff, black dots on scalp, favus (yellow crusts, matted hair), and kerion. *Tinea pedis* is an environmental skin disorder of the toe web that is acquired either through a contact with infected skin or by a fungus in the environment. High prevalence of *Tinea pedis* has been reported in schoolchildren: 12% in the United Kingdom, 16.9% in Israel, 5.2% in Australia, and 7.8% in Peru. The diagnosis of superficial dermatomycoses can be confirmed by a dermoscopic examination or culture. Avoiding direct skin-to-skin contact with infected individual and improving personal hygiene are among measures that reduce the risk of contamination.

Keywords Dermatomycosis · Pityriasis versicolor · Tinea capitis · Tinea pedis

---

N. R. Ngatu, M.D., Ph.D.
Graduate School of Medicine, International University of Health and Welfare (IUHW), Chiba, Japan

Graduate School of Public Health, International University of Health and Welfare (IUHW), Tokyo, Japan

N. R. Ngatu, M. Ikeda (eds.), *Occupational and Environmental Skin Disorders*,
https://doi.org/10.1007/978-981-10-8758-5_11

List of Abbreviations

BCH	Bar code-like hair
CH	Coma hair
CSH	Corkscrew hair
EFSD	Environmental fungal skin disease
ZH	Zigzag hair

11.1 Background

11.1.1 Definition of Dermatomycoses

Dermatomycoses are fungal diseases of the skin. Dermatophytes are infectious agents that have keratinase and cause infection in the keratinized human and animal tissues such as the skin, hair, and nail to cause a disease known as dermatophytosis (Molina de Diego 2011). Environmental fungal skin disorders (EFSD) have a worldwide distribution, with high prevalence in most developing countries.

11.1.2 Etiology and Risk Factors for Environmental Dermatomycoses

11.1.2.1 Etiology of Dermatomycoses

Common dermatomycoses are caused by dermatophytes (Table 11.1) and opportunistic fungi: *Malassezia*, *Candida*, *Trichosporon*, *Rhodotorula*, *Cryptococcus* or *Aspergillus*, *Geotrichum*, *Alternaria*, etc. When considering their primary habitat of the fungal agents, they are divided into three types:

- "Anthropophilic" dermatophytes: they are parasitic organisms that infect humans.
- "Zoophilic" dermatophytes: those that infect animals.
- "Geophilic" dermatophytes: they are fungi found in the soil.

There are approximately several species of dermatophytes, of which 40 species belonging to the genera *Epidermophyton*, *Trichophyton*, and *Microsporum* (Molina de Diego 2011). The present paper focuses on common prevalent dermatomycoses in human subjects and their causative agents.

11.1.2.2 Risk Factors of Dermatomycoses

Based on previous reports, it has been established that EFSD evolve along with predisposing and associated factors such as:

- Environmental and geographical factors (climate, humidity)
- Human factors (population mobility, personal hygiene, abusive antifungal drug use)

- Economic factor (poverty)

These factors determine disease distribution in regions of the world. For example, *Trichophyton violaceum*, *Trichophyton verrucosum*, and *Microsporum ferrugineum* are reported to be endemic in some African, Asian, and European countries, whereas *Trichophyton rubrum*, *Trichophyton interdigitale*, *Trichophyton tonsurans*, and *Microsporum canis* are getting more frequent globally (Zhang and Liu 2017).

Table 11.1 Common anthropophilic dermatophytes and their geographical distribution (Modified from Nenoff et al. 2014a, b)

Dermatophyte species	Localization	Observation
Trichophyton rubrum	Most common dermatophyte worldwide; *Trichophyton rubrum* var. *raubitschekii* is found mainly in Africa but has also been isolated in Germany, Turkey, Spain, and Japan	It causes *Tinea pedis, tinea unguium*, and *tinea corporis T. rubrum* Is the most common cause of *tinea pedis* (athlete's foot) in sub-Saharan Africa
Trichophyton tonsurans	Found in America, Africa, and Asia	It causes tinea capitis
Trichophyton violaceum	It is found mainly in Africa	It is the most prevalent dermatophyte in Africa
Trichophyton soudanense	It is found in Africa	It shares the same genotype with *Trichophyton violaceum*
Trichophyton schoenleinii	It is rarely found in Europe but quite common in other continents	–
Trichophyton megninii	It is found in Europe (British countries)	It causes *T. pedis*, *T. unguium*, *T. barbae*, and *T. manuum*
Trichophyton mentagrophytes var. *interdigitale*	It is found in Europe and North America	They cause *tinea unguium* or fungal nail infection, resulting in a red, itchy, scaly, circular rash
Trichophyton concentricum	It is found in Southeast Asia	It causes *tinea imbricata*
Epidermophyton floccosum	It is can be found worldwide	It causes *T. pedis* and *T. corporis*
Microsporum audouinii	It is mainly found in the sub-Saharan African region	It causes tinea capitis in some countries in the Caribbean
Microsporum ferrugineum	This dermatophyte is most common in the far east, Korea, northern China, Thailand, Japan, the Middle East, and Nigeria (Raina et al. 2016)	It causes *T. corporis*
Microsporum canis	It is a cosmopolite dermatophyte	It causes tinea capitis in dogs and cats, hamsters, and lions and also easily contaminates humans, children in particular

11.2 Tinea Capitis

11.2.1 Definition and Epidemiology

T. capitis is a mycosis of the scalp (Fig. 11.1). It is reported to be the most prevalent dermatomycosis in childhood in several countries of the world. It is mainly caused by the dermatophytes *T. tonsurans* and *M. audouinii*. In Europe, *M. canis*, a zoophilic dermatophyte, remains the most common causative agent of *T. capitis* (Elghblawi 2017; Ginter-Hanselmayer et al. 2007). Prevalence rate of *T. capitis* differs according to geographic regions of the world. Rates of 2.5% in London (Hay et al. 1996), 0.1% in Germany (Mohrenschlager et al. 2005), 0.3% in Italy (Polonelli et al. 1982), 7.1% in Tanzania, and 31.2% in Nigeria (Perez-Gonzalez et al. 2009)

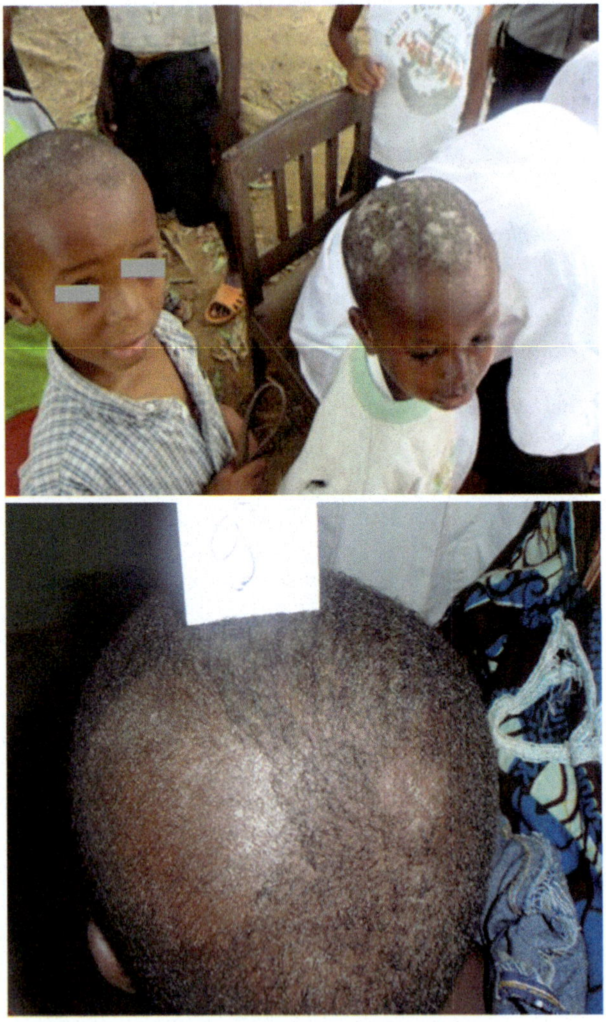

Fig. 11.1 Tinea capitis in Congolese schoolchildren taken care during the "Mobile Clinic Project" in Kongo Central province, Democratic Republic of Congo, 2011 (photo by the authors) Risk Factors and Prevention of T. Capitis

have been reported. A 30-year retrospective hospital-based survey in southern Spain on dermatomycoses diagnosed between 1977 and 2006 found 818 cases of which 444 (54%) were *T. capitis* cases (del Boz et al. 2011).

In the Unites States (US), *T. capitis* prevalence rate of 3–8% has been reported, whereas in the sub-Saharan African region, relatively higher rates of this disease can be found in the literature: 50–56% in Ethiopia, 7.1% in Tanzanian schools, and 7.4% in Egypt (Faergemann et al. 2006), and, in our previous school-based study, 11.2% of Congolese primary and junior high schoolchildren with skin disorders had *T. capitis* (Ngatu et al. 2011).

11.2.2 Clinical Manifestations and Diagnosis

The clinical diagnosis of *T. capitis* can be thought of in the presence of:

- Dry scaling-like dandruff usually with moth-eaten hair loss
- Black dots (hairs are broken off at the scalp surface)
- Favus (yellow crusts and matted hair)
- Kerion (inflamed mass like an abscess)

In addition, the presence of dermoscopic (trichoscopic) features (Table 11.2) that characterize the disease, such as coma hair (CH), zigzag hair (ZH), Morse code or bar code-like hairs (BCH), and/or corkscrew hair (CSH), in white patient should lead the healthcare provider to consider the diagnosis of *T. capitis* (Fig. 11.2).

Table 11.2 Proposed clinical diagnostic criteria for *T. capitis*

Clinical feature (Trichoscopic marker)	Definition	Observation
Coma hairs (CH)	First described *T. capitis* clinical feature, it represents cracking of hair shafts	Not specific to *T. capitis*, but it is a feature of dermatophytosis of the scalp in darker skin
Zigzag hair (ZH)	Due to its structural weakness as the dermatophyte perforates the hair cuticle and causes the hair to bend	–
Morse code-like hairs or bar code-like hairs (BCH) (Lin and Li 2014; Elghblawi 2017)	The presence of irregularly interrupted hairs with normal pigmentation and paler narrowed intervals. Infected hair appears as empty bands related to localized areas of infection	–
Corkscrew hair (CSH) (Neri et al. 2013)	It is a hair type that is fragile and breaks easily; it is often pale, transparent, or gray (in adult white in particular) and may result in alopecia	CSH can also be found in other skin conditions (copper deficiency, malnutrition)

Notes: The table was made by authors using information provided by Neri et al. (2013), Lin and Li (2014), and Elghblawi (2017)

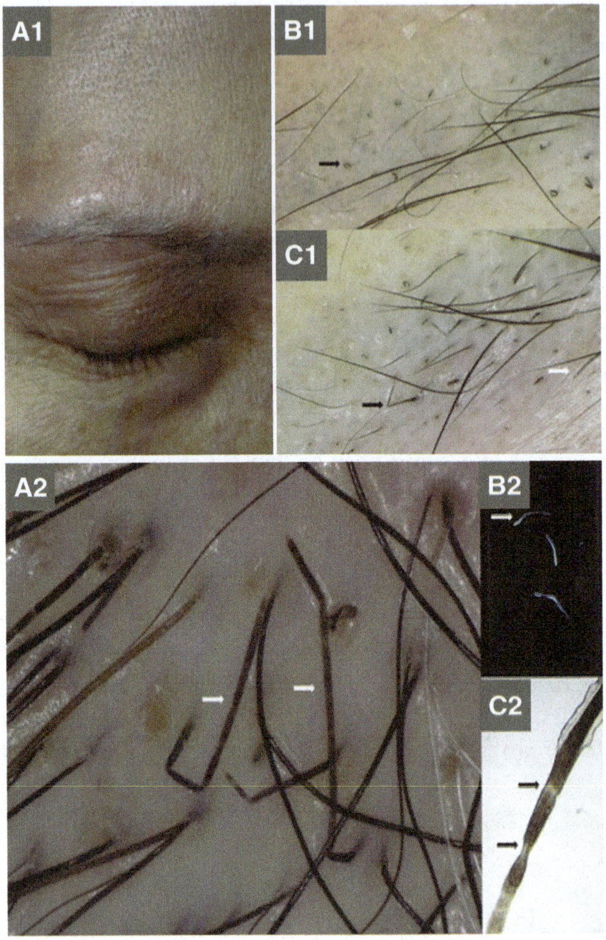

Fig. 11.2 Patient 1. (**A1**) Image showing the patient with a 3.5 cm × 4.5 cm round erythematous patch with fine scaly borders and reduced density of her right eyebrow. (**B1**) Dermoscopy of the right lateral eyebrow showed comma hairs (black arrow, magnification 6x). (**C1**) Dermoscopy of the right medial eyebrow showed zigzag hair with bar code-like features (black arrow) and bar code-like hairs (white arrow, magnification 6x). Patient 2: (**A2**) Dermoscopy revealed diffuse bar code-like hairs, zigzag hairs (white arrows), comma hair, black dots, and broken hairs (magnification 6x). (**B2**) Three plucked hairs including a bar code-like hair (white arrow) showed green fluorescence under the Wood's lamp. (**C2**) The bar code-like hair was examined under the microscope, which showed that the paler or hypopigmented parts were also narrower (black arrows) (magnification 10x) (©2013 Elsevier Taiwan LLC, Permission to reuse from editors, Dermatologica Sinica; Lin and Li 2014)

However, to confirm the diagnosis, laboratory investigations are of great importance, for example, microscopy and the culture of skin craping. The major complications and sequelae of *T. capitis* are intense pruritus, bacterial infection, and alopecia.

School settlement has been reported to be the main risk factor for *T. capitis.* (Balci et al. 2014). Other factors are also associated with this skin condition:

- Poor hygiene
- Age
- Overcrowding
- Use of shared combs
- Ethnicity
- Hairdressing salons
- In order to prevent the disease, the following steps can be of help, particularly in groups at risk:
- Shampooing the hair regularly
- Avoidance of sharing combs, clothes, and other items (headgear, soap, towel) to prevent the spread of the infection
- Have pets examined by an animal doctor
- Improved general personal hygiene

11.3 Tinea Pedis (Athlete's Foot)

11.3.1 Definition and Epidemiology

Tinea pedis or athlete's foot is a common environmental fungal infection that occurs in the interdigital toe web space as well as the skin of the feet (Fig. 11.3). It is caused by some of the species of fungal agents or dermatophytes, namely, *Trichophyton* spp. (*T. rubrum*, *T. mentagrophytes*, and *Epidermophyton floccosum*); they are said to be the most frequent agents identified. Previous reports have suggested *Microsporum* as another cause (Brooks and Bender 1996; Bell-Syer et al. 2012; Kaushik et al. 2015). Any part of the foot can be affected by *T. pedis*, and the same fungal agents can affect the nails (onychomycosis) and hands. The disease is typically acquired either through a contact with infected skin or by a fungus in the environment, and *T. pedis* can also spread from animals (Bell-Syer et al. 2012; Moriarty et al. 2012). Athlete's foot is a prevalent skin disorder in several regions of the world. Globally, *T. pedis* affects approximately 15% of the population. It occurs most frequently in older children and young adult, with males being most affected than females (Kaushik 2015). High prevalence has been reported in schoolchildren population: 12% in the United Kingdom, 16.9% in Israel, 5.2% in Australia, 7.8% in Peru, 0.15%–2% in Turkey, and 2.5% in Spain (Moriarty et al. 2012; Balci et al. 2014).

11.3.2 Clinical Manifestations, Complications, and Diagnosis

In addition to pruritus (itching) and redness, scaly lesions and blisters (severe cases) are often seen on the patient's foot. *T. pedis* comprises three clinical forms: interdigital, plantar (moccasin foot), and vesiculobullous. Of those forms, interdigital is

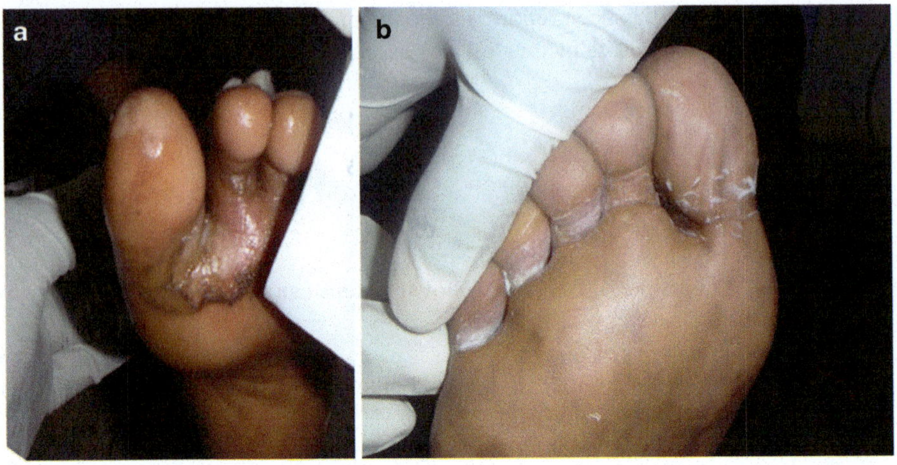

Fig. 11.3 Tinea pedis in an adult Congolese patient complicated with bacterial infection (**a**) and another T. pedis patient who was recovering (having a few skin lesions on fourth and fifth toes) under topical ketoconazole treatment (**b**), "Mobile clinic project 2011", Kongo Central, Democratic Republic of Congo (photo by the authors)

the most common clinical manifestation that is characterized by maceration and fissuring of the skin mainly in the space between the toes, whereas plantar *T. pedis* is characterized by hyperkeratotic plaque and squamous plaques that cover the soles, heels, and sides of the foot (Toukabri et al. 2017).

In a patient presenting with *T. pedis* clinical manifestations (see above), the diagnosis can be confirmed either by culture or seeing hyphae using a microscope. The most common complication is bacterial infection, which is characteristic of the severe form of the disease. The disease can also cause other dermatomycosis such as *T. unguium.*

11.3.3 Risk Factors and Preventive Measures

Factors such as the use of occlusive shoes, occupations requiring vigorous physical activity, and wet conditions have been reported to be the main risk factors of fungal infections of the foot. In Brazil, Sabadin et al. (2011) reported that having familial cases of fungal infection and contact with domestic animals were risk factors for dermatomycosis of the foot. A recent study by Picardo-Geisinger et al. (2014) found that Latino immigrants who always or most of the time use occlusive shoes had a higher prevalence of developing either *T. pedis* or *onychomycosis* as compared to other ethnic groups.

A study conducted by Toukabri et al. (2017) in northern Africa (Tunisia) has found that main predisposing factors of *T. pedis* were the practice of ritual washing and the frequentation of communal showers, accounting for 56.6% and 50.5%, respectively. A number of measures have been proposed for athlete's foot (Kaushik et al. 2015); they include:

- Avoiding to walk barefoot in public showers
- Changing socks daily
- Wearing big enough shoes
- Avoid sharing shoes, sandals, etc.
- Keeping toenails short
- Avoid sweating the feet

When already infected by *T. pedis* agent:

- Keep the feet dry and clean
- Wear sandals

11.4 Pityriasis (or Tinea) Versicolor

11.4.1 Definition and Etiology of P. Versicolor

Pityriasis or tinea versicolor is one of common noninflammatory superficial cutaneous fungal infections caused by lipophilic fungi, *Malassezia* yeasts (*M. furfur*, *M. globosa*, *M. sympodialis*), characterized by changes in skin pigmentation (Fig. 11.4). It is also known as dermatomycosis furfuracea and tinea flava. Adults are the most affected, but the disease is also common in schoolchildren from tropical areas (Schwartz 2004, Rai and Wankhande 2009; Dioussé et al. 2017).

Predisposing factors of P. versicolor are as follows:

1. Heat
2. Occlusion
3. Depressed cellular immunity
4. Moisture (Park et al. 2010)

11.4.2 Epidemiology, Clinical Manifestations, and Diagnosis of P. Versicolor

P. versicolor has a worldwide distribution; however, its frequency varies depending on climatic, socioeconomic, and occupational conditions. In Iran, the disease represents 6% of all skin diseases and approximately 30% of dermatomycoses (Sunenshine et al. 1998). Prevalence as high as 50% has been found in tropical countries. In Sweden, a survey showed a 0.5% of P. versicolor (Renati et al. 2015).

Malassezia species produce chemicals known as dicarboxylic acids (e.g., azelaic acid) that inhibit tyrosine kinase, resulting in hypopigmentation of the skin area involved. In other individuals, hyperchromic or erythematous lesions may also appear. Skin symptoms comprise oval-shaped or rounded dyschromic maculas in seborrheic areas (Erchiga and Florencio 2002; Dias et al. 2013).

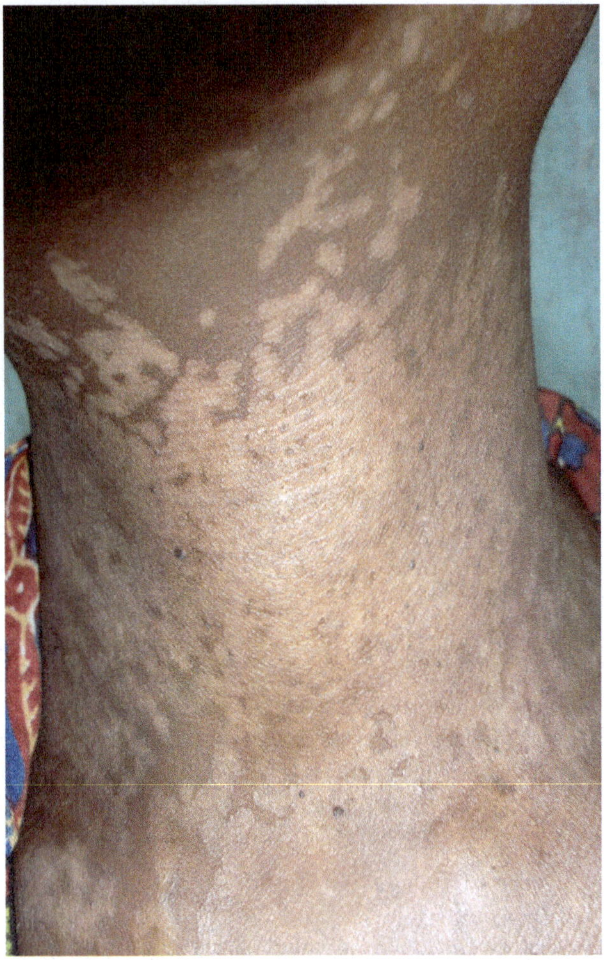

Fig. 11.4 A 24-year-old Congolese girl with tinea versicolor skin lesions (dyschromic macules) on the neck and upper chest (photo from authors; Mobile clinic project 2011, Kongo central, DR Congo)

The diagnosis can be made based on clinical features of skin lesions but a confirmation established by detecting hyphae and spores with a direct laboratory examination with the use of potassium hydroxide.

11.4.3 Risk Factors and Preventive Measures for P. Versicolor

Factors such as poor hygiene, immunodepression, sweating, malnutrition, heat, and humidity can contribute to the occurrence of T. versicolor. On the other hand, a number of measures can be applied to prevent the occurrence and the spread of the disease:

1. Good hygiene
2. Avoidance of contact with infected persons
3. Avoidance of sharing of hygiene articles and clothes
4. Application of measures to avoid immune suppression

11.5 Other Environmental Dermatomycoses

Tinea unguium: it is a mycosis of the nails caused mainly by *T. rubrum*, *T. mentagrophytes* var. *interdigitale*, and *E. floccosum*.

Tinea cruris: it often occurs in patients with tinea pedis or onychomycosis, caused by *T. rubrum*, *T. mentagrophytes* var. *interdigitale*, and *E. floccosum*. Predisposing factors are diabetes, obesity, and sweating.

Candidiasis: it is caused by *Candida albicans* and other *Candida* types (*C. parapsilosis*, *C. tropicalis*, *C. stellatoidea*, etc.). Exposed occupations and groups are as follows: maids, dishwashers, cooks, nurses, and elderly. Nails and folds (interdigital, inframammary, axillary, ungual) can be affected.

Tinea corporis and *tinea manuum*.

11.6 Treatment of Dermatomycoses

Superficial fungal infections (mycoses) can be easily treated when a correct diagnosis is established and a good treatment choice is made. However, in individuals with immunosuppression, a severe form of the disease often occurs, requiring more potent antifungal agents (Tampieri 2004). Below, we present different antifungal agents used in the management of dermatomycosis (Table 11.3).

Table 11.3 Systemic and topical treatment for dermatomycoses (based on Dias and Quaresma-Santos 2013)

Disease	Medication (drug)
Tinea capitis	• *systemic treatment:* – *Griseofulvin* (micronized: 20–25 mg/kg/day for 6–12 weeks; ultramicronized drug, 10–15 mg/kg/day for 6–12 weeks) – *Terbinafine* (7 mg/kg/day for 6 weeks) – *Itraconazole* (5 mg/kg/day for 6 weeks) – *Fluconazole* (8 mg/kg/day for 8 weeks)
Pityriasis versicolor	• *systemic treatment:* – *Ketoconazole* (200 mg/day for 10 days) – *Fluconazole* (200 mg/day for 7 days) – *Itraconazole* (200 mg/day for 7 days)
Tinea pedis	• *systemic treatment:* – *Terbinafine* (oral: 200 mg 2 times/day for 1 week) – *Itraconazole* (oral: 200 mg 2 times/day for 1 week) – *Fluconazole* (oral: 150 mg once/week for 2–4 weeks) – *Ketoconazole* (oral: 200–400 mg/day for >4 weeks) – *Griseofulvin* (oral: Micronized 1 g/day; ultramicronized 660–750 mg/day for 4–8 weeks) • *topical treatment:* – *Terbinafine* (cream, 1–2 applications a day for 1–4 weeks, or 1% solution, 1–2 applications a day for 1 week) – *Ketoconazole* (2% cream: 1 application/day for 6 weeks) – *Ciclopirox* (0.77% cream: 2 applications/day for 4 weeks)

11.7 Conclusion

Environmental fungal skin disorders are common diseases worldwide. The correct diagnosis and, eventually, the identification of the causative fungal agent are imperative for a good disease management. More importantly, the implementation of preventive measures and appropriate treatment of patients are crucial to prevent or limit further spread of environmental dermatomycoses.

References

Balci E, Gulgun M, Babacan O, et al. Prevalence and risk factors of tinea capitis and tinea pedis in schoolchildren in Turkey. J Pak Med Assoc. 2014;64(5):514–8.

Bell-Syer SE, Khan SM, Torgerson DJ. Oral treatments for fungal infections of the skin of the foot. Cochrane Database Syst Rev. 2012;17:10. https://doi.org/10.1002/14651858.CD003584.pub2.

del Boz J, Crespo V, Rivas-Ruiz F, de Troya M. A 30-year survey of paediatric tinea capitis in southern Spain. J Eur Acad Ermatol Venereol. 2011;25(2):170–4.

Brooks KE, Bender JF. Tinea pedis: diagnosis and treatment. Clin Podiatr Med Surg. 1996;13(1):31–46.

Dias MFRG, Quaresma-Santos MVP, Bernades-Filho F, et al. Update on therapy for superficial mycoses: review article part I. An Bras Dermatol. 2013;88(5):764–74.

Dioussé P, Ly F, Bammo M, et al. Pityriasis versicolor in newborn children: unusual clinical aspects and role of depigmentation in mother (French article). Pan Afr Med J. 2017;26:31.

Elghblawi E. Tinea capitis and trichoscopic criteria. Int J Trichology. 2017;9(2):47–9.

Erchiga VC, Florencio VD. Malassezia species in skin diseases. Curr Opin Infect Dis. 2002;15(2):133–42.

Faergemann J, Ausma J, Borgers M. The *in vivo* activity of R126638 and hetoconazole against *Malassezia* species. Acta Derm Venereol. 2006;86:312–5.

Ginter-Hanselmayer G, Weger W, IIkit M, Smolle J. Epidemiology of tinea capitis in Europe: current state and changing patterns. Mycoses. 2007;50(2):6–13.

Hay RJ, Clayton YM, De Silva N, et al. Tinea capitis in south-East London-a new pattern of infection with public health implications. Br J Dermatol. 1996;135:955–8.

Kaushik N, Pujalte GG, Reese ST. Superficial fungal infections. Prim Care. 2015;42(4):501–16.

Lin YT, Li YC. The dermoscopic coma, zigzag, and bar code-like hairs: markers of fungal infection of the hair follicles. Dermatol Sin. 2014;32(3):160–3.

Mohrenschlager M, Bruckbauer H, Seidl HP, et al. Prevalence of asymptomatic carriers and cases of tinea capitis in five to six-year-old preschool children from Augsburg, Germany: results from the MIRIAM study. Pediatr Infect Dis. 2005;24:749–50.

Molina de Diego A. Clinical diagnostic and therapeutic aspects of dermatophytosis (article in Spanish). Enferm Infecc Microbiol Clin. 2011;29(3):33–9. https://doi.org/10.1016/S0213-005X(11)70025-8.

Moriarty B, Hay R, Morris-Jones R. The diagnosis and management of tinea. BMJ. 2012;345(7):e4380.

Nenoff P, Kruger C, Hanselmayer GH, Tietz HJ. Mycology—an update. Part 1: dermatomycoses: causative agents, epidemiology and pathogenesis. J Dtsch Dermatol Ges. 2014a;12(3):188–209. https://doi.org/10.1111/ddg.12245.

Nenoff P, Kruger C, Schaller J, et al. Mycology—an update part 2: dermatomycoses: clinical picture and diagnosis. J Dtsch Dermatol Ges. 2014b;12(9):749–77. https://doi.org/10.1111/ddg.12420.

Neri I, Starace M, Patrizi A, Balestri R. Corkscrew hair: a trichoscopy marker of tinea capitis in an adult white patient. JAMA Dermatol. 2013;149(8):990–1.

Ngatu NR, Saruta T, Hirota R, Eitoku M, Muzembo BA, Matsui T, et al. Antifungal efficacy of Brazilian green propolis extracts and honey on Tinea capitis and Tinea versicolor. Eur J Integr Med. 2011;3:e281–7.

Park HJ, Lee YW, Cho YB, et al. Skin characteristics in patients with Pityriasis Versicolor using non-invasive method, MPA5. Arch Dermatol. 2010;146(10):1132–40.

Perez-Gonzalez M, Torres-Rodriguez JM, Martinez-Roig A, et al. Prevalence of tinea pedis, tinea unguium of toenails and tinea capitis in school children from Barcelona. Rev Iberoam Micol. 2009;26:228–32.

Picardo-Geisinger R, Mora DC, Newman JC, et al. Comorbidity of tinea pedis and onychomycosis and evaluation of risk factors in Latino immigrant poultry processing and other manual laborers. South Med J. 2014;107(6):374–9.

Rai MK, Wankhande S. Pityriasis versicolor-an epidemiology. J Microbial Biochem Technol. 2009;1:051–6.

Raina D, Gupta P, Khanduri A. A first case of Microsporum ferrugineum causing tinea coproris in Uttarakhand. Annals Trop Med Public Health. 2016;9(5):351–3.

Renati S, Cukras A, Bigby M. Pityriasis versicolor. BMJ. 2015;350:h1394.

Sabadin CS, Benvegnu SA, da Fontoura MM, et al. Onychomycosis and tinea pedis in athletes from the state pf Rio Grande Do Sul (Brasil): a cross-sectional study. Mycopathologia. 2011;171(3):183–9.

Schwartz RA. Superficial fungal infections. Lancet. 2004;364(9440):1173–82.

Sunenshine PJ, Schwartz RA, Janniger CK. Tinea versicolor: an update. Cutis. 1998;61:65–8.

Tampieri MP. Update on the diagnosis of dermatophytosis. Parasitologia. 2004;46(1–2):183–6.

Toukabri N, Dhieb C, El Euch D, et al. Prevalence, etiology and risk factors of Tinea pedis and Tinea unguium in Tunisia. Can J Infect Dis Med Microbiol. 2017;2017:6835725.

Zhang P, Liu W. The changing face of dermatophytic infections worldwide. Mycopathologia. 2017;182(1–2):77–86. https://doi.org/10.1007/s11046-016-0082-8.

Chapter 12
Sarcoptic Skin Disease (or Scabies)

Roger Wumba and Nlandu Roger Ngatu

Abstract Sarcoptic skin disease (SSD), also called scabies or "itch mite," is a cosmopolite itchy and contagious ectoparasitic infection of the skin caused by *Sarcoptes scabiei* var. *hominis*. According to the World Health Organization (WHO), SSD affects approximately 300,000,000 people annually, mostly in developing countries. In Asia, very high SSD prevalence rate has been reported in Australian aboriginal population, reaching up to 50%, and in the Pacific Rim islands such as Fiji (18.5%), Vanuatu (24%), and Solomon Islands (25%). Crowded houses and schools, poor hygiene, reduced access to medical or nursing care, and faulty application of treatment agents are among risk factors of SSD. Recent works have proposed the sero-diagnostic approach for scabies, consisting of the detection of *Sarcoptes scabiei* protein tyrosine kinase (SsPTK), which is similar to PTK from rabbit ear mite *Psoroptes ovis cuniculi* and widely distributed at the front end of the *Sarcoptes* mite, legs, and mouthparts with the use of an indirect ELISA. Another novel diagnostic approach being studied consists of the use of immunofluorescence staining technique. Researchers found a novel inorganic pyrophosphatase Ssc-PYP-1 located in the tegument around the mite's mouthparts, the cuticle, and the entire legs and then developed an indirect ELISA using recombinant Ssc-PYP-1 (rSsc-PYP-1) as the capture antigen to diagnose sarcoptic mite in naturally infected mammals, with high sensitivity and specificity, 92% and 93.6%, respectively. Raising awareness and providing financial support to program aiming at SSD control and elimination are among measures to be implemented to reduce global SSD burden.

Keywords Itch mite · *Sarcoptes scabiei* · Sarcoptic skin disease · Protein tyrosine kinase

R. Wumba, M.D., Ph.D.
Department of Tropical Medicine, Faculty of Medicine, University of Kinshasa, Kinshasa, Congo

N. R. Ngatu (✉)
Graduate School of Medicine, International University of Health and Welfare (IUHW), Chiba, Japan

Graduate School of Public Health, International University of Health and Welfare (IUHW), Tokyo, Japan

N. R. Ngatu, M. Ikeda (eds.), *Occupational and Environmental Skin Disorders*,
https://doi.org/10.1007/978-981-10-8758-5_12

Abbreviations

CI	Confidence interval
CNS	Central nervous system
N	Number
WHO	World Health Organization
OR	Odd ratio
SSD	Sarcoptic skin disease
SsPTK	*Sarcoptes scabiei* tyrosine kinase

12.1 Introduction

12.1.1 Definitions of Sarcoptic Skin Disease (Scabies)

Sarcoptic skin disease (SSD) is a cosmopolite itchy and contagious ectoparasitic infection of the skin caused by *Sarcoptes scabiei* var. *hominis*. SSD has been a health problem for humans since the first millennium; it spreads rapidly in human communities in the event of defective hygiene and promiscuity (Fédération Wallonie-Bruxelles 2013; Canadian Pediatric Society 2001). SSD patients are often subject to persisting stigmatization, prejudices, bullies, or teases (Oustric 2014). It is a dermatitis that is widespread all over the world irrespective of climate and affects both men and women of all ages and socioeconomic backgrounds (Gaspard et al. 2013).

In industrialized countries, SSD usually manifests by epidemics affecting particular institutions such as hospitals, daycare centers, kindergarten, etc., whereas in middle- and low-income countries, it is endemic particularly in tropical and subtropical countries, thus representing a real public health issue (Oustric 2014; Heukelbach and Feldmeier 2006) (Fig. 12.1).

12.1.2 Epidemiologic Profile and Risk Factors for SSD

The World Health Organization (WHO) has declared SSD a "neglected disease" (Feldmeier and Heukelbach 2009); it affects approximately 300,000,000 people annually, mostly in low-income countries where 50% of the population can be infected during epidemics (Nair et al. 1977; Gaspard et al. 2013; Demarest 2015). In the United States, data from health insurance registries of workers from the private sector, covering over 5,000,000 workers and their families, indicated a SSD incidence of 68.8 cases/100,000 per year between 2001 and 2005 (Haut Conseil de Santé Publique 2012).

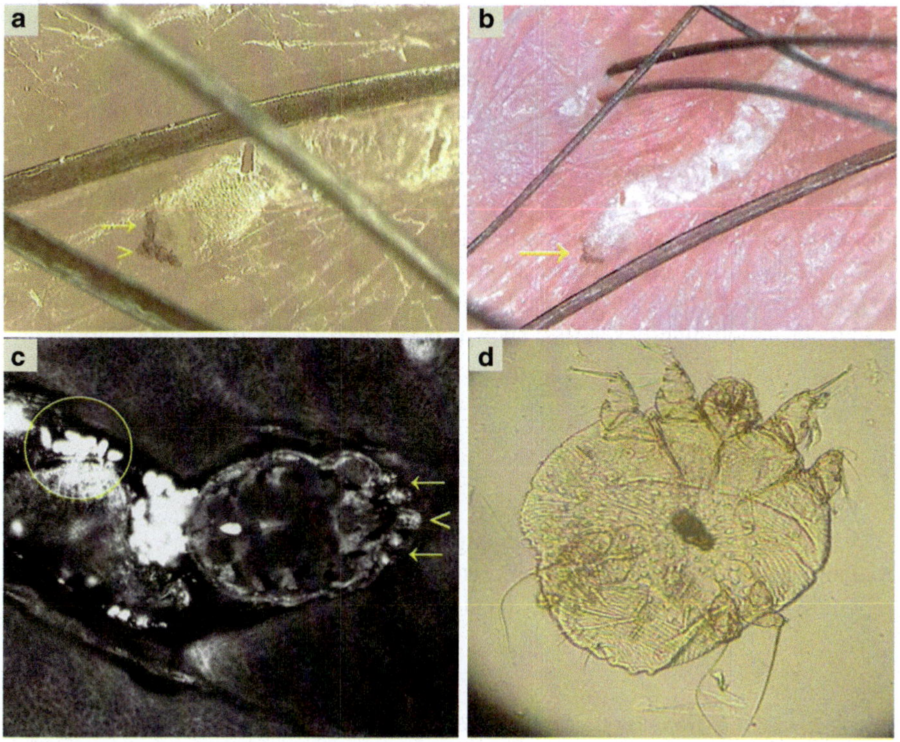

Fig. 12.1 (**a–d**) *Sarcoptes scabiei* var. *hominis* figure (**a**) shows Sarcoptes scabiei observed by videodermatoscopy at 400× magnification; the mite, localized at the end of the burrow, has a roundish body and pigmented head (arrowhead) and anterior legs (arrow). Figure (**b**) shows a skin area affected by scabies observed using a low-cost video microscope at 150× magnification. Both the burrow and the mite (arrow) are clearly evident. Figure (**c**) shows a Sarcoptes scabiei observed at the end of a burrow by handheld confocal microscopy, with a technique that enables a detailed visualization of the head (arrowhead) and of the anterior legs (arrows); the feces appear as high-refractive roundish structures (circle) [© Micali et al. 2016, PlosOne]. Figure (**d**) shows the image of Sarcoptes scabiei (Photocredit: ©Kalumet via Wikimedia Commons https://creativecommons.org/licenses/by-sa/3.0/legalcode)

In Europe, SSD rates vary according to countries. Higher SSD incidence has been reported in France, 328 cases/100,000 per year between 2005 and 2009, and authors have suggested an increasing disease incidence in this country. In Belgium, a comprehensive study conducted in 2004 that included general practitioners, dermatologists, and pediatricians from the city of Ghent has shown an incidence of 28 cases/100,000 per year but with a response rate very low (4%) among the surveyed doctors in Great Britain (Haut Conseil de Santé Publique 2012). On the other hand, in the British countries, health registry records (for the period between 1971 and 2003) of two samples of 60 and 91 doctors showed that the number of consultations for SSD was 370, 120, 340, 470, and 233 consultations per 100,000 per year in

1971, 1981, 1991, 2000, and 2003, respectively (Haut Conseil de Santé Publique 2012).

In Asia, high SSD prevalence has been reported among young people in rural India (70%) (Nair et al. 1977) and in Australian aboriginal populations (up to 50%) (Carapetis et al. 1997). Similarly, relatively high rates of this skin disorder have been found in schoolchildren populations in the Pacific Rim islands such as Fiji (18.5%), Vanuatu (24%), and the Solomon Islands (25%) (Carapetis et al. 1997). In the African continent, previous studies have shown disparities in prevalence rates of SSD (Heukelbach and Feldmeier 2006; Hegab et al. 2015; Kouotou et al. 2016).

A number of risk factors have been reported to facilitate the occurrence SSD outbreaks in communities at risk, such as poor, rural, or aboriginal populations:

- High pediatric population density
- Lack of running water
- Crowded housing, shared beds
- Crowded schools
- Failure to recognize an infestation
- Reduced access to medical or nursing care
- Failure to eradicate scabies from clothing and bed linen
- Faulty application of treatment agents

12.2 Transmission of *Sarcoptes scabiei* Disease and Clinical Manifestations

During infestation, *Sarcoptes scabiei* burrows into the epidermis, between the *stratum corneum* and Malpighian layer; it does not penetrate into the dermis. SSD symptoms include skin inflammation, itching, vesicles and crusty skin lesions. Indigenous and impoverished people are the most vulnerable populations (Heukelbach and Feldmeier 2006; Shen et al. 2017). Pruritus appears mostly 3–4 weeks after the occurrence of infestation. It is not directly related to the presence of the parasite, but reactions of hypersensitivity from antigens of adults, eggs and excreta sensitizing the immunocompetent cells in the dermis.

Overnight, itch can be the cause of insomnia. Initially, it is located at interdigital spaces, and then it is quickly spreading to the wrists, the ulnar, and the hands and then at the elbows, armpits, nipples, abdominal, and inguinal region. After a few days, it is widespread. In addition, nodules and a hyperkeratosis develop, most frequently in the elderly and immunocompromised individuals. SSD skin lesions mainly localized on the upper (hands, interdigital spaces, wrist, elbow, armpit) and lower (foot, interdigital spaces of feet, ankle, knee) limbs, buttocks, chest, and genital organs (Figs. 12.2 and 12.3). Because of the possibility to find scabies' lesions on the genital organ, the disease has been considered as a sexually transmitted illness.

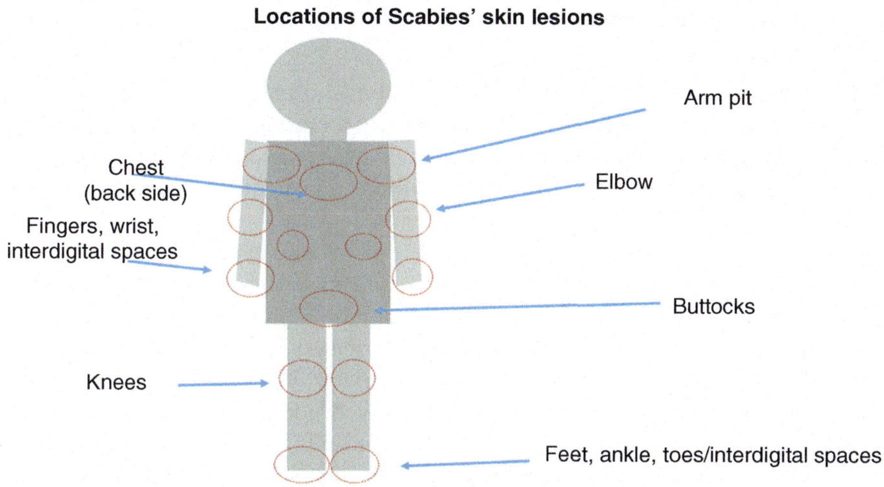

Fig. 12.2 Possible locations of Sarcoptes scabiei disease's skin lesions on the body surface (Source: authors)

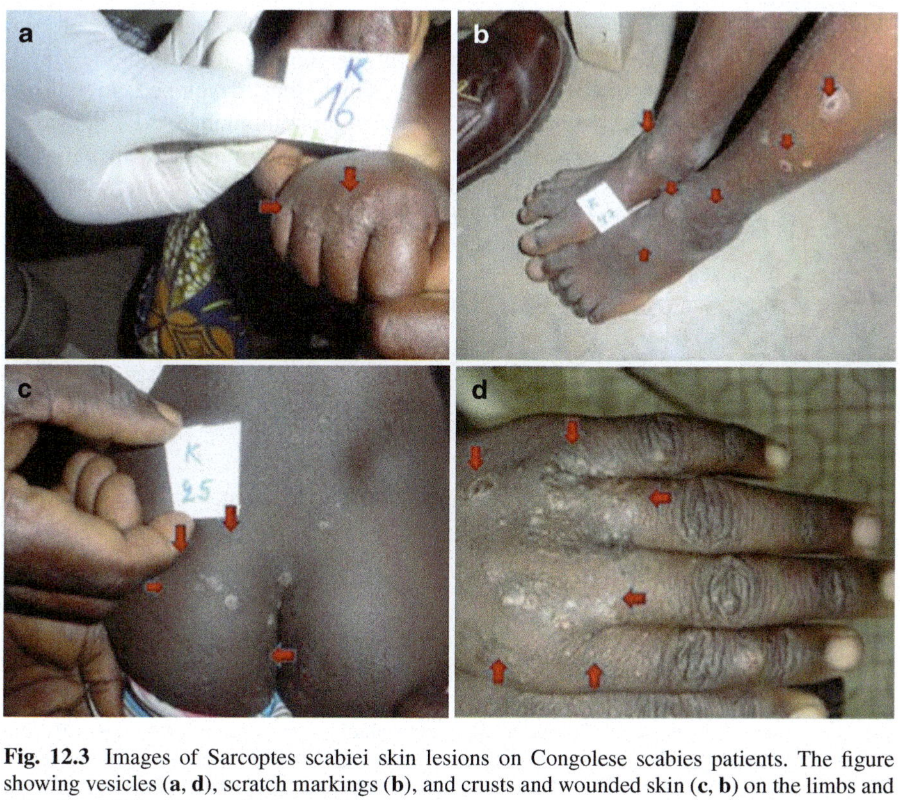

Fig. 12.3 Images of Sarcoptes scabiei skin lesions on Congolese scabies patients. The figure showing vesicles (**a**, **d**), scratch markings (**b**), and crusts and wounded skin (**c**, **b**) on the limbs and buttocks of SSD patients (Source: authors)

12.3 Diagnostic Approach

SSD diagnosis is mainly clinical, based on patient's disease history and skin symptoms. Night pruritus can be evocative of disease topography. The confirmation of SSD can be done through direct parasitological examination after skin scraping on affected region. The use of a dermoscope allows to visualize the mites (Nair et al. 1977).

Recently, a novel research proposed a serodiagnostic approach that consists of the detection of *Sarcoptes scabiei protein tyrosine kinase* (SsPTK), a ~30 kDa protein that shares high homology with a PTK from the rabbit ear mite *Psoroptes ovis cuniculi* (Shen et al. 2017). SsPTK is widely distributed at the front end of *Sarcoptes* mite, in the chewing mouthparts and legs particularly. Shen et al. (2017) found that indirect ELISA using recombinant SsPTK showed good diagnostic value (95.2% sensitivity and 94.1% specificity) for detecting anti-PTK antibody in serum samples of infested rabbits (Fig. 12.4). Additionally, PTK ELISA could diagnose SSD in the early stages of the infection with an accuracy of 100%. This suggests that SsPTK has a potential to serve as a sensitive antigen for the early diagnosis of parasitic mite infestation.

In addition, Xu et al. (2017) proposed a new diagnostic approach for scabies. With the use of immunofluorescence staining technique, they found a novel inorganic pyrophosphatase Ssc-PYP-1, located in the tegument around the mite's mouthparts, the cuticle, and the entire legs. Then, they developed an indirect enzyme-linked immunosorbent assay (ELISA) using recombinant Ssc-PYP-1 (rSsc-PYP-1) as the capture antigen in order to diagnose sarcoptic mite in naturally infected mammals (rabbits). The assay had high sensitivity (92% and specificity (93.6%), suggesting that it could be an efficient laboratory serodiagnostic procedure

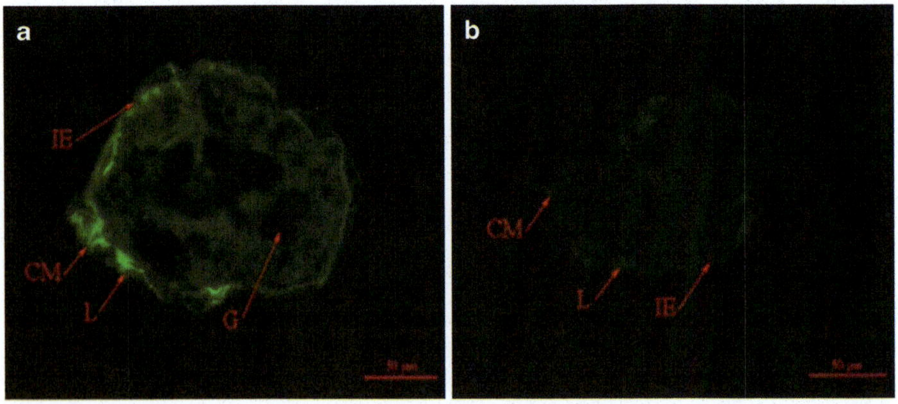

Fig. 12.4 Immunolocalization of PTK in Sarcoptes scabiei tissue; (**a**) staining with anti-PTK as the primary antibody, (**b**) negative control [© Shen et al. 2017; http://creativecommons.org/licenses/by/4.0/. No change was made]. *IE* epidermal integument; *CM* chewing mouthpart; *L* leg; *G* gut

for scabies in newly infected animals; this study also provides insight on the possibility to develop similar SSD diagnosis in human subjects.

12.4 Complications of Sarcoptic Skin Disease

(a) *Infections*: mostly, those infectious skin disorders are superficial. They include: impetigo and cellulitis. However, those infections may generalize and cause impetigo, sepsis, glomerulonephritis, chronic renal (kidney) disease, rheumatic arthritis which may lead to rheumatic heart disease (Engelman et al. 2013).
(b) *Other complications*: complicated SSD includes eczematous skin diseases, lichenification, and crust formation on the skin of infected individuals.

12.5 Management of Sarcoptic Skin Disease

The treatment of SSD or scabies in infested patients consists of the administration of anti-SSD medication to the patient and people surrounding him (Nair et al. 1977; Shen et al. 2017). Drugs currently in use comprise *permethrin* (it is reported to be the most effective medication), *lindane*, *crotamiton*, *benzyl benzoate*, *ivermectin*, *malathion*, and *sulfur* (Walker and Johnstone 2000). *Ivermectin* derived from *avermectin*, a drug developed by Dr. Omura and Dr. Cambell who are winners of The 2015 Nobel Prize in Physiology/Medicine. The US Center for Disease Control and Prevention (CDC), the WHO, and the International Union against Sexually Transmitted Infections have proposed guidelines for the management of scabies (Table 12.1).

Currently, SSD global control measures are being promoted. They include three main priorities:

- Raising awareness of scabies and financial support
- Enhancing clinical and epidemiologic study for a better understanding of SSD
- Development and implementation of effective control strategies (Engelman et al. 2013)

Table 12.1 Guidelines for the treatment of ordinary scabies

Guidelines	Recommended regimens	Alternatives
CDC (division: sexually transmitted diseases prevention)	• *Permethrin:* apply once for 8–14 h • *Ivermectin:* 200 μg/kg on day 0 and 2 weeks later (oral administration; but its safety in pregnant women and young children not established yet)	• *Lindane*: apply once for 8 h, day 0, and 2 weeks later
WHO/International Union against sexually transmitted infections)	• *Permethrin:* apply once for 8–12 h • *Ivermectin:* 200 μg/kg on day 0 and 2 weeks later • *Sulfur:* apply for 3 days	• *Benzyl benzoate:* apply for 2–3 consecutive days

Notes: This table is based on report from Khalil et al. (2017)

12.6 Conclusion

SSD is a contagious disease that is transmitted either by direct, prolonged skin-to-skin contact with an infested person or through sexual contact. Thus, avoiding skin-to-skin contact with an infested individual or with items such as clothing or bedding that is used by an individual affected by SSD is one of the best ways to prevent contamination. Additionally, household members and other potentially exposed persons (schoolmates, siblings, etc.) should be treated at the same time as the infested person to prevent possible reexposure and reinfestation.

References

Canadian Pediatric Society. Scabies management. Paediatr Child Health. 2001;6(10):775–7.
Carapetis JR, Connors C, Yarmirr D, et al. Success of a scabies control program in an Australian aboriginal community. Pediatr Infect Dis J. 1997;16:494–9.
Demarest MR. La gale en recrudescence en France: point de vue des médecins généralistes et attitude thérapeutique lors de la prise de la gale en cabinet de médecine générale, Thèse Présentée à la Faculté de médecine Henri Warebourg de l'Université Lille 2 Droit et Santé, Lille, 2015.
Engelman D, Kiang K, Chosidow O, et al. Toward the global control of human cabies: introducing the international alliance for the control of scabies. PLoS Negl Trop Dis. 2013;7(8):e2167.
Fédération Wallonie-Bruxelles. Sarcoptes skin disease (French article). 2013. http://www.federation-wallonie-bruxelles.be/index.php?id=gale. Accessed Dec 2013.
Feldmeier H, Heukelbach J. Epidermal parasitic skin diseases: a neglected category of poverty-associated plagues. Bull World Health Organ. 2009;87:152–9.
Gaspard L, Laffitte E, Eicher N et al., Prise en charge de la gale: généralités sur la gale, Hôpitaux Universitaires de Genève, AH/NE/EL Mars 2013 (published in French) 2013.
Haut Conseil de Santé Publique (HCSP). Communicable diseases: Recommendations on the management of one or more cases of Scabies; 2012 Report, France (Report in French). http://www.hcsp.fr/explore.cgi/avisrapportsdomaine?clefr=313.
Hegab DS, Kato AM, Kabbash IA, et al. Scabies among primary schoolchildren in Egypt: socio-medical environmental study in Kafr el-sheikh administrative area. Clin Cosmet Investig Dermatol. 2015;8:105–11.
Heukelbach J, Feldmeier H. Scabies. Lancet. 2006;367:1767–74.
Khalil S, Abbas O, Kibbi AG, et al. Scabies in the age of increasing drug resistance. PLoS Negl Trop Dis. 2017;11(11):e0005920.
Kouotou EA, Nansseu JRN, Kouawa MK, et al. Prevalence and drivers of human scabies among children and adolescents living and studying in Cameroonian boarding schools. Parasit Vectors. 2016;9:400.
Micali G, Lacarrubba F, Verzì AE, et al. Scabies: advances in noninvasive diagnosis. PLoS Negl Trop Dis. 2016;10(6):e0004691.
Nair BK, Joseph A, Kandamuthan M. Epidemic scabies. Indian J Med Res. 1977;65:513–8.
Oustric E. La gale sarcoptique humaine: maladie, épidémiologie, diagnostic, traitements et prise en charge à l'officine, Thèse présentée à la faculté des sciences pharmaceutiques de l'Université de Toulouse III Paul Sebatier, Toulouse, 2014.
Shen N, He R, Liang Y, et al. Expression and characterization of Sarcoptes scabiei protein tyrosine kinase as a potential antigen for scabies diagnosis. Sci Rep. 2017;7(1):9639. https://doi.org/10.1038/s41598-017-10326-w.

Walker GJ, Johnstone PW. Interventions for treating scabies. Cochrane Database Syst Rev. 2000;3:CD000320.

Xu J, Huang X, He M, et al. Identification of a novel PYP-1 gene in Sarcoptes scabiei and its potential as a serodiagnostic candidate by indirect-ELISA. Parasitology. 2017:1–10. https://doi.org/10.1017/S0031182017001780.

Chapter 13
Frequency and Clinical Features of Sarcoptic Skin Disease (Scabies) in Congolese Schoolchildren

Wumba Roger and Nlandu Roger Ngatu

Abstract Sarcoptic skin disease (SSD) or scabies is a contagious parasitic skin disorder caused by the acarine itch mite *Sarcoptes scabiei* var. *hominis. SSD is prevalent in the developing world where* outbreaks occur in mostly vulnerable communities and health institutions, resulting in a significant economic burden. The World Health Organization (WHO) has estimated a SSD global prevalence of 0.2–24%. In Africa, relatively high SSD rates have been reported in children populations: 7.7–8.3% in remote areas in Kenya, 10.5% in Nigeria, and 17.8% in rural Cameroon. We conducted a cross-sectional descriptive study that included schoolchildren from four primary schools in Kinsenso, a semi-urban county of Kisenso in Kinshasa, Democratic Republic of Congo (DRC). Clinical examination was undertaken to diagnose and determine the frequency of SSD among schoolchildren. Ethical approval and necessary authorizations were obtained. Results showed a SSD rate of 3.95% in the population of Congolese schoolchildren (N1 = 2024) and 3.4% in a sample of those with skin disorders (N2 = 1894). The majority of affected children were boys (56% vs. 44% for girls). Personal hygiene was defective in 80% of participants. The younger children (5–7 years) were the most affected (61.5%); interdigital spaces were found to be the most affected body parts (93.8%), and vesicle was the most frequent skin lesion (95.3%). SSD represents a public health issue in DRC, and preventive measures should be implemented for SSD control and, eventually, its eradication.

Keywords Democratic Republic of Congo · Epidemiology · *Sarcoptic skin disease* · Scabies · Schoolchildren

---

W. Roger
Department of Tropical Medicine, Faculty of Medicine, University of Kinshasa, Kinshasa, Congo

Faculty of Medicine, William Booth University, Kinshasa, Congo

N. R. Ngatu, M.D., Ph.D. (✉)
Graduate School of Medicine, International University of Health and Welfare (IUHW), Chiba, Japan

Graduate School of Public Health, International University of Health and Welfare (IUHW), Tokyo, Japan

N. R. Ngatu, M. Ikeda (eds.), *Occupational and Environmental Skin Disorders*,
https://doi.org/10.1007/978-981-10-8758-5_13

Abbreviations

DRC Democratic Republic of Congo
SSD Sarcoptic skin disease
WHO World Health Organization

13.1 Background

13.1.1 Definition and Epidemiologic Profile of Scabies

Sarcoptic skin disease (SSD) or scabies is a contagious parasitic skin disorder caused by the acarine itch mite *Sarcoptes scabiei* var. *hominis*. *It is a prevalent dermatosis in the developing world where* outbreaks occur mostly in vulnerable communities and health institutions, resulting in a significant economic burden. SSD also represents a major public health problem in indigenous populations in Australia, with a prevalence reaching 25% in adults and 30–65% in children (Andrews et al. 2009; Heukelbach et al. 2013). The World Health Organization (WHO) estimates SSD global prevalence to be 0.2–24% (WHO 2005; Thomas et al. 2016).

In Africa, epidemiologic surveys have shown varying prevalence of SSD. In Egypt, a cross-sectional study conducted among primary schoolchildren from Kafr El Sheikh area showed prevalence rate of 4.4% (Hegab et al. 2015). Recently, Kouotou et al. (2016) found a prevalence rate of 17.8% among children living in boarding schools in Cameroon. In southern Ethiopia, a prevalence rate of 5.5% was recently observed (Walker et al. 2017). To our knowledge, there have been no scientific reports on SSD in Congolese schoolchildren.

13.1.2 Rationale and Study Objectives

The purpose of this study was to determine the epidemiologic profile of SSD in schoolchildren at a suburban Kisenso county in Kinshasa, Democratic Republic of Congo (DRC). Its objectives were as follows:

- To determine the frequency of SSD in schoolchildren population in suburban area of Kisenso in Kinshasa, Democratic Republic of Congo (DRC), more specifically the proportion of SSD schoolchildren in the sample of children with skin disorders at the time of this study
- To determine the sociodemographics of Congolese SSD schoolchildren
- To determine the clinical features and complications of SSD in Congolese schoolchildren from suburban county of Kisenso
- To investigate the role played by bodily and dressing hygiene in the occurrence of SSD in Congolese schoolchildren

13.2 Material and Methods

13.2.1 Study Sites and Population

This was a cross-sectional descriptive study conducted in randomly selected four schools in the semi-urban "Mission county" in Kisenso area in Kinshasa, DRC, from September 1 to November 2015. A list of all schools of the Kisenso county was obtained from administrative authorities from which four schools were randomly selected: Saint Achille school (781 students), Genious of Kisenso school (629 students), Kayila school (588 students), and Rehoboth school (206 students), making up a population of 2204 schoolchildren.

13.2.2 Study Sample

The study sample was drawn from the population of schoolchildren from four selected schools. Inclusion criteria were as follows:

1. Being a student at one of the selected schools
2. Being present at school at the time of enrollment

A total of 2204 children were enrolled; of them, 1894 (85.9%) presented with cutaneous symptoms related to skin disorders.

13.2.3 Clinical Examination

After receiving approvals from local health zone authority and school headmasters, we proceeded with the recruitment of study participants. A patient form was used for each participant to anonymously collect information on sociodemographics and on which data from the clinical examination were recorded. The clinical examination consisted of the description of the types and locations of skin lesions on the body (interdigital, hand, face, elbow, axillary, abdominal folds, inguinal folds, genital area). In addition, information on bodily and dressing hygiene, as well as current treatment, was also recorded.

13.2.4 Ethical Considerations

The study protocol was approved by the local health zone authority and accepted by the directors of all participating schools. The handling of study data during data collection, their transcription on registration forms, and analysis was performed anonymously, and confidentiality was assured in regard to the privacy of study participants. None of procedures undertaken during the study could cause harm to the participants, and all related activities were carried out in conformity with the Helsinki declaration on the use of human subjects in research.

13.2.5 Data Analysis

Collected data were transcribed on an Excel sheet using Excel 97-2003 software and analyzed with the use of Epi info software version 2007.

13.3 Results

13.3.1 Frequency of Sarcoptes scabiei (SSD) Disease Among Schoolchildren

The mean age of the study participants was 7.75 ± 2 years (range: 5–13 years). SSD rate was 3.4% (75/2204) in the sample of enrolled schoolchildren and 3.95% (75/1894) in those with skin disorders. Table 13.1 presents SSD prevalence according to gender, age group, and school in Kisenso area. Scabies were more frequent in male schoolchildren than in females, 60% and 40%, respectively, for a sex ratio of 1.5. When age was considered, the majority of SSD schoolchildren were aged 5–7 years, followed by the age group 8–10 years (27.69%) and 11–13 years (10.76%). We then compared SSD prevalence according to school, and it was found that SSD was more frequent at Saint Achille school (4.85%, 36/741), followed by

Table 13.1 Rate and clinical features of SSD among schoolchildren with skin disorders

Characteristics	Confirmed SSD ($N = 75$)	%
Gender		
M ($n = 1137$)	42	56
F ($n = 757$)	33	44
Age group (year)		
5–7	40	61.53
8–10	18	27.69
11–13	17	10.76
School		
Saint Achille ($n = 741$)	36	4.85
Kisenso Genious ($n = 590$)	14	2.37
Kayila ($n = 367$)	8	2.17
Rehoboth ($n = 196$)	7	3.57

Rehoboth school (3.57%, 7/196) and Kisenso Genious school (2.37%, 14/590) and Kayila school (2.57%, 8/367) (Table 13.1).

Physical examination of SSD schoolchildren revealed a number of signs and symptoms. It was found that vesicles were the most prevalent skin lesions in SSD schoolchildren, representing 95.38% of all clinical manifestations. They were followed by scratching markings, 4.61%. Pruritus (itch) and furrows had a low frequency, 1.53% (not shown).

13.3.2 Location of Scabies' Lesions in Infested Schoolchildren

Table 13.2 shows the distribution of main skin lesions on body parts. It was found that 93.84% of schoolchildren had SSD skin lesions in interdigital spaces. On the other hand, the anterior wrist and ulnar border of the hands were the second prevalent locations of scabies in schoolchildren who participated in this study.

13.3.3 Body Location of Scabies' Lesions in Infested Schoolchildren

Table 13.3 shows different complications that occurred in SSD schoolchildren. The results revealed that the majority (82.8%) had no complication, 11.42% had scratching lesions, 4.28% had infectious complication (impetigo), and 1.42% developed eczema.

Table 13.2 Frequency (%) distribution of skin lesions according to their localization

Location of SSD lesions	Frequency (*n*)	%
Interdigital spaces	**61**	**93.84**[#]
Anterior wrist surface	11	16.92
Ulnar border of the hands	11	16.92
Armpits	**6**	9.23
Male genital organs	**6**	9.23
Elbows	**1**	1.53
Nipples	**9**	13.84
Abdominal folds	**5**	7.69
Inguinal folds	**9**	13.84

[#]*p*-value less than 0.001

Table 13.3 Frequency (%) distribution of scabies complications in schoolchildren

Scabies complications	Frequency (*n*)	%
Scratching lesions	8	11.42
Impetigo lesions of scalp	3	4.28
Eczematous lesions	1	1.42
No complications	58	82.85

13.3.3.1 Personal Dressing Hygiene Status in Schoolchildren and Treatment Used Against Scabies' Cutaneous Clinical Manifestations

Regarding personal dressing hygiene, a markedly higher proportion (80%, 52/65) of schoolchildren had a defective dressing hygiene (vs. acceptable dressing hygiene group, 20%; $p < 0.01$). However, there was no significant difference when considering the gender (Fig. 13.1a) and age group (Fig.13.1b) of the study participants. Moreover, no association was observed between personal dressing hygiene and SSD in schoolchildren.

Table 13.4 shows different treatment options used to treat SSD schoolchildren. It reveals that a large majority (83%) of SSD schoolchildren did not receive any medication, whereas only approximately 7.69% of patients received appropriate anti-SSD medication and 1.53% received ethnomedical remedies.

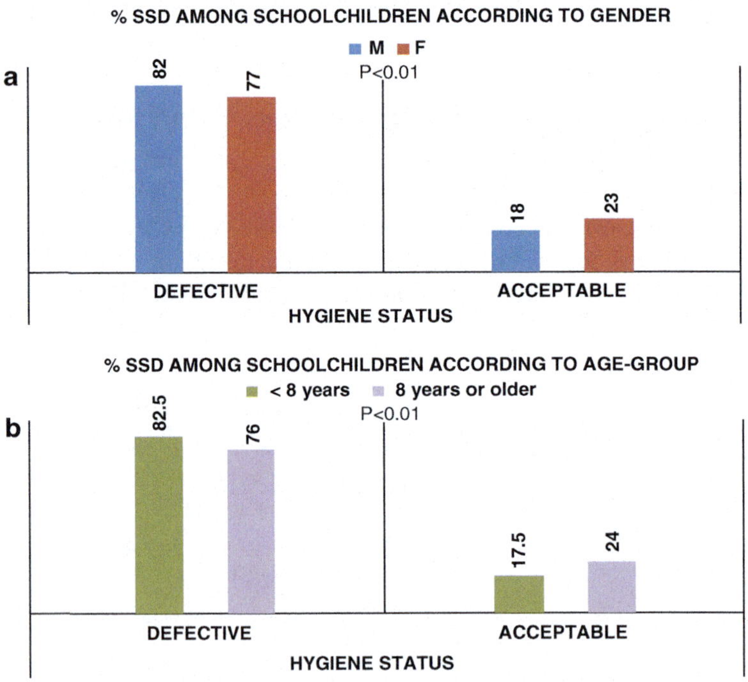

Fig. 13.1 (**a**, **b**) Proportion of scabies-affected schoolchildren with defective or acceptable personal dressing hygiene according to gender (**a**) and age group (**b**). Figure shows that there were more schoolchildren with defective dressing hygiene (vs. acceptable hygiene, $p < 0.01$) and no significant difference when comparing male vs. female SSD schoolchildren in terms of dressing hygiene status. Similarly, no significant difference was noted when comparing younger (<8 years of age) vs. older (8 years or older) schoolchildren

Table 13.4 Therapeutic approaches used by SSD children

Type of therapy	*N* (65)	%
Anti-SSD cream	5	7.69
Ethnomedical remedies	1	1.53
Others (ignored)	5	7.69
No medication	54	83.07

SSD sarcoptes scabiei disease, *N* number of cases, % percentage

13.4 Discussion

The present study determined the frequency of SSD in a sample of 1894 schoolchildren with skin disorders from Kisenso semirural county in Kinshasa, DRC. The majority of affected children were boys. The most affected schoolchildren had younger age (5–7 years); interdigital spaces were found to be the location with higher proportion of SSD skin lesions (93.8%), and vesicle was the most frequent skin lesion (95.3%). Personal hygiene was defective in 80% of schoolchildren, and more than half of SSD schoolchildren were not under any anti-scabies medication at the time of this study.

The frequency of SSD found in this study (3.95% in the study sample and 3.4% in the study population) is low compared to reports from other African studies. Higher SSD prevalence (8.3% and 7.7%) has been reported in Kenya (8.3% and 7.7%) (Schmeller and Dzikus 2001), in Nigeria (10.5%) (Kalu et al. 2015), and recently in Cameroon (17.8%) (Kouotou et al. 2016). In addition, our study showed that male schoolchildren were the most affected; this fact has also been reported previously in Mali (Landwehr et al. 1998). Furthermore, several studies have shown higher prevalence of SDD in younger schoolchildren. For example, Tounkara (1994) in Mali found that schoolchildren aged 10–14 years were the most affected, and our study showed a higher frequency of SSD in schoolchildren aged 5–7 years. The fact that SSD is often common in young children can be explained by the tendency of this category of children to have defective dressing hygiene, particularly in remote African towns and villages and also in communities where poverty is rampant.

A relationship between poverty and SSD and also between overcrowding (close personal contact) and SSD has been reported in previous works (Currie et al. 1994, McCarthy et al. 2004). DRC is one of the countries where extreme poverty is rampant and schools in most remote areas are overcrowded; thus, outbreaks of poverty-related diseases are quite recurrent and even endemic. Moreover, the lack of anti-scabies treatment that was observed in over 80% of SSD schoolchildren might be one of factors that might have contributed to the spread of the disease in those schools. Nevertheless, this study has a limitation. The cross-sectional design of this study suggests that its findings are true for participating schools and may not reflect the real situation of SSD in Congolese schools. Future research projects that include more schools from both remote and urban areas should be envisaged.

13.5 Conclusion

The aim of this pilot study was to contribute to the improvement of pediatric SSD management. Although it was undertaken in a semi-urban area, this study shed light on the epidemiology and clinical manifestations of SSD among Congolese schoolchildren. In addition, results from this study may serve to elaborate appropriate strategies for the prevention and control of this ectoparasitosis which has obvious health, cognitive, social, and psychological consequences.

Findings from this study may also serve as base for future investigations on risk factors, sociologic and anthropologic perceptions of Congolese populations toward SSD in Kinshasa, the control of *Sarcoptes* mites, and appropriate therapeutic agents for SSD. Additionally, more emphasis should be put on contamination of humans and the disease prevention during community health interventions. Furthermore, anti-SSD educational campaigns for the general population, social and community leaders, and the general population should be implemented to increase awareness.

References

Andrews RM, Keams T, Connors C, et al. A regional initiative to reduce skin infections amongst aboriginal children living in remote communities of the Northern territory, Australia. PLoS Negl Trop Dis. 2009;3:e554.

Currie BJ, Connors CM, Krause VL. Scabies programs in aboriginal communities. Med J Aust. 1994;161:636–7.

Hegab DS, Kato AM, Kabbash IA, et al. Scabies among primary schoolchildren in Egypt: socio-medical environmental study in Kafr el-sheikh administrative area. Clin Cosmet Investig Dermatol. 2015;8:105–11.

Heukelbach J, Mazigo HD, Ugbomoiko US. Impact of scabies in resource-poor communities. Curr Opin Infect Dis. 2013;26:127–32.

Kalu EI, Wagbatsoma V, Ogbaini-Emovon E, et al. Age and sex prevalence of infectious dermatoses among primary school children in a rural south-eastern Nigerian community. Pan Afr Med J. 2015;20:182.

Kouotou EA, Nansseu JRN, Kouawa MK, et al. Prevalence and drivers of human scabies among children and adolescents living and studying in Cameroonian boarding schools. Parasit Vectors. 2016;9:400.

Landwehr D, Keita SM, Pönnighaus JM, Tounkara C. Epidemiologic aspects of scabies in Mali, Malawi, and Cambodia. Int J Dermatol. 1998;37(8):588–90.

McCarthy JS, Kemp DJ, Walton SF. Scabies: more than just an irritation. Postgrad Med J. 2004;80:382–7.

Schmeller W, Dzikus A. Skin diseases in children in rural Kenya. Br J Dermatol. 2001;144:118–24.

Thomas J, Carson CF, Peterson GM, et al. Therapeutic potential of tea tree oil for scabies. Am J Trop Med Hyg. 2016;94(2):258–66.

Tounkara C. Clinical, epidemiologic and therapeutic aspects of scabies in Bamako (PhD thesis published in French). Ecole Nationale de Médecine et de Pharmacie du Mali, 1994. http://www.keneya.net/fmpos/theses/1993/pdf/93M10.pdf.

Walker SL, Lebas E, De Sario V, et al. The prevalence and association with health-related quality of life of tungiasis and scabies in schoolchildren in southern Ethiopia. Plos Negl Trop Dis. 2017;11(8):e0005808.

World Health Organization (WHO). Epidemiology and management of common skin diseases in children in developing countries. Geneva, Switzerland: WHO; 2005. http://whqlibdoc.who.int/hq/2005/WHO_FCH_CAH_05.12_eng.pdf?ua.

Chapter 14
Paederus Dermatitis: Environmental Risk Factors, Clinical Features, and Management

Nlandu Roger Ngatu

Abstract Paederus dermatitis (spider lick, night burn, blister beetle dermatitis, or dermatitis linearis) is a form of irritant contact dermatitis (ICD) that is characterized by a sudden onset of erythematobullous lesions on exposed body areas. This skin disorder is caused by a beetle of the genus *Paederus*. A number of environmental factors have been reported to be associated with Paederus dermatitis, including artificial lights, crop harvest, and dispersal of Paederus beetles and climate influence. Skin lesions and symptoms develop within 6–48 h after a contact with *pederin*, a toxic substance that is released after crushing the insect against the body; they include skin burning and stinging (generally precede other symptoms), itching, erythematous plaques, edema, vesicles, and/or blisters. Paederus dermatitis can be prevented by applying a series of measures such as avoidance of sitting under artificial light sources during seasons of P. dermatitis outbreaks, avoidance of crushing Paederus beetle against the skin (blow it off instead of crushing it), closing doors and windows at night during the season of outbreak, careful use of insecticides to reduce Paederus beetle population in the living environment (but avoid contamination of the environment), removal of vegetation near residential buildings and houses, and the use of light sources that less attract insects, if possible. Washing the affected body area with soap and clean water and the application of cold wet compresses, after skin contact with *pederin*, may reduce the risk of developing skin lesions. On the other hand, an oral antibiotherapy can be envisaged in case of infection.

Keywords Irritant contact dermatitis · Paederus dermatitis · Paederus beetle · Prevention

N. R. Ngatu, M.D., Ph.D.
Graduate School of Medicine, International University of Health and Welfare (IUHW), Chiba, Japan

Graduate School of Public Health, International University of Health and Welfare (IUHW), Tokyo, Japan

N. R. Ngatu, M. Ikeda (eds.), *Occupational and Environmental Skin Disorders*,
https://doi.org/10.1007/978-981-10-8758-5_14

Abbreviation

ICD Irritant contact dermatitis

14.1 Background: Definition and Epidemiology of Paederus Dermatitis

14.1.1 Definition and Overview on Paederus Dermatitis Outbreaks

Paederus dermatitis (spider lick, night burn, blister beetle dermatitis, or dermatitis linearis) is a form of irritant contact dermatitis (ICD) that is characterized by a sudden onset of erythematobullous lesions on exposed body areas. This skin disorder is caused by a beetle of the genus *Paederus*. The insect does not sting or bite its victims but releases a toxic fluid known as *pederin*. The dermatitis occurs after human skin contact (mainly neck and face) with *pederin* (Sendur et al. 1999; Mammino 2011; Nasir et al. 2015). Member of the Staphylinidae family, the genus *Paederus* has about 622 species with a worldwide distribution; of them, a number of species are reported to cause the dermatitis in humans: *P. sabaeus* in Central Africa region, *P. fuscipes* in the Middle East and South America, *P. melampus* in India, and *P. colombius* and *P. brasiliensis* in South America (Arnold et al. 1990; Nasir et al. 2015; Bazrafkan et al. 2016).

Paederus beetle is relatively slender and can be easily identified; the adult insect is 1.5 mm wide and 7–10 mm long, with a black head and red or orange thorax (Frank and Kanamitsu 1987). Outbreaks of Paederus dermatitis have occurred in many countries of the world, including Australia, Malaysia, Okinawa (Japan), Nigeria, Sierra Leone, Kenya, Uganda, Brazil, Argentina, Venezuela, Ecuador, France, India, etc. (Sing and Yousuf Ali 2007).

14.1.2 Paederus Dermatitis Outbreaks in Central Africa Region

Compared to the Southeast Asia and South America, the Central Africa region is the most affected region by seasonal outbreak of a dermatitis caused by *P. sabaeus*. In the region, countries that are close to the equator (Democratic Republic of Congo, Republic of Congo, Central Africa Republic) experience annual regional epidemic during the period preceding the dry season, between April and May. Several thousands of people are affected in each of these countries. However, the epidemic remains underreported.

One of the first reports from the Central Africa region consisted on P. dermatitis outbreaks that occurred in Brazzaville, the capital of the Republic of Congo; in Kinshasa, the capital of the Democratic Republic of Congo (DRC); in Libreville, the capital of Gabon; and in Bangui, the capital of Central Africa Republic, in the year 1993 (Penchenier et al. 1994). Similar outbreaks have occurred in the 1970s. This can be understood as most Central African cities started using electric power in those years. The first reported Brazzaville epidemic occurred at the beginning of May 1993, when the first cases were admitted at a local hospital; and on May 15, 1993, almost all the city was affected. From two to three beetles found around electric lamps, the number reached hundreds of Paederus beetles and remained constant until the end of May 1993. At the same period, cases of P. dermatitis were observed in Bangui and Franceville (Gabon).

In DRC, epidemics of *P. sabaeus*-caused dermatitis occur both in urban and rural cities, and almost all households are affected, irrespective of economic and social statuses. The most recent scientific report from DRC consisted of an unusual widespread outbreak among Indian troops serving in the United Nations' Peace Force in DRC between 2007 and 2008. The epidemic occurred not in April or May but between September 2007 and March 2008. In total, 154 clinically diagnosed cases of P. dermatitis were registered, including military personnel of male Indian origin aged 22–36 years (Vasudevan and Joshi 2010), with a peak of the dermatitis (121 cases) between mid-October to mid-December 2007. All patients noticed P. dermatitis skin lesions for the first time after waking up in the morning, and they presented with skin burning feeling over the lesions. Most lesions (vesicles, erythematous halo; the characteristic "kissing lesion" was found only in two patients) were located on exposed body parts (71.8%) such as forearms (27%), and most patients had multiple skin lesions (47.4%). The majority of patients responded well to topical sulfadiazine, whereas patients with scrotum and periorbital involvement did not tolerate mupirocin treatment. Residual hyperpigmentation persisted for 4–8 weeks.

14.2 Environmental Factors Associated with Paederus Dermatitis

Paederus dermatitis affects people of all ages and social statuses, given that this skin condition does not depend neither on occupation nor people's activities. Nighttime contact with the insect is very common. Occupational exposure to Paederus beetle may also occur during the day. Their most common habitat is crop fields, but they can also be found in riverbanks and marshes; they migrate from their habitat to humans' living environment for different reasons. Factors that are reported to be associated with Paederus dermatitis are as follows:

- *Artificial lights*: Paederus beetles are attracted to sources of indoor lights and light towers that increase the beetles' migration to residential areas.

- *Crop harvest and dispersal of Paederus beetles*: the elimination of their habitat during harvest processes forces Paederus beetles to move from croplands to humans' living environment. A recent study by Maryam et al. (2016) showed that bright light source and high altitude (elevation of buildings or residences) were main factors that attract Paederus beetles, causing them to disperse, invade human shelters, and cause outbreaks of P. dermatitis. These phenomena coincide with the period of rice and corn harvest according to regions of the world.
- *Climate or seasonal influence*: climate has a direct effect on activities of Paederus beetles, and outbreaks of Paederus dermatitis occur during the rainy season and during hot and humid weather. However, in some regions, epidemics occur after the rainy season when temperatures rise, suggesting that Paederus beetles might seek indoor shelters to escape extreme weather outdoor (Markgraf and Basedow 2002; Lima et al. 2015).

14.3 Clinical Features, Histopathological Changes, and Complications of Paederus Dermatitis

After a skin contact with the toxic substance (*pederin*) from Paederus beetle's (Fig. 14.1a) body, the onset of symptoms is often delayed 6–48 h after exposure. Most common symptoms of Paederus-caused dermatitis linearis are:

- Burning and stinging (generally precede other symptoms)
- Itching
- Erythematous plaques and edema (Fig. 14.1b–d)
- Vesicles and/or blisters

The vesicles (blisters) may turn into pustules. Some patents report having unexplained skin lesions or itching, suggesting that they accidentally crushed the insect while sleeping (Sing and Yousuf Ali 2007; Beaulieu and Irish 2016).

The primary histopathological change that occurs in the course of the disease is a neutrophilic spongiosis that leads to a vesiculation and a reticular epidermal degeneration. The neutrophilic infiltration with confluent necrosis and the reticular degeneration represent the main pathological characteristics of Paederus dermatitis. On the other hand, acanthosis, parakeratosis that contains neutrophilic exudate, can be seen in older skin lesions (Banney et al. 2000).

The differential diagnosis should be established by considering other skin disorders that have similar clinical features. Paederus dermatitis can easily be confused with allergic or irritant contact dermatitis, photodermatitis, fungal skin infections, herpes zoster and herpes simplex, bullous impetigo, and pustular psoriasis (Sujit and Koushik 1997; Beaulieu and Irish 2016). The main complication of P. dermatitis is infection.

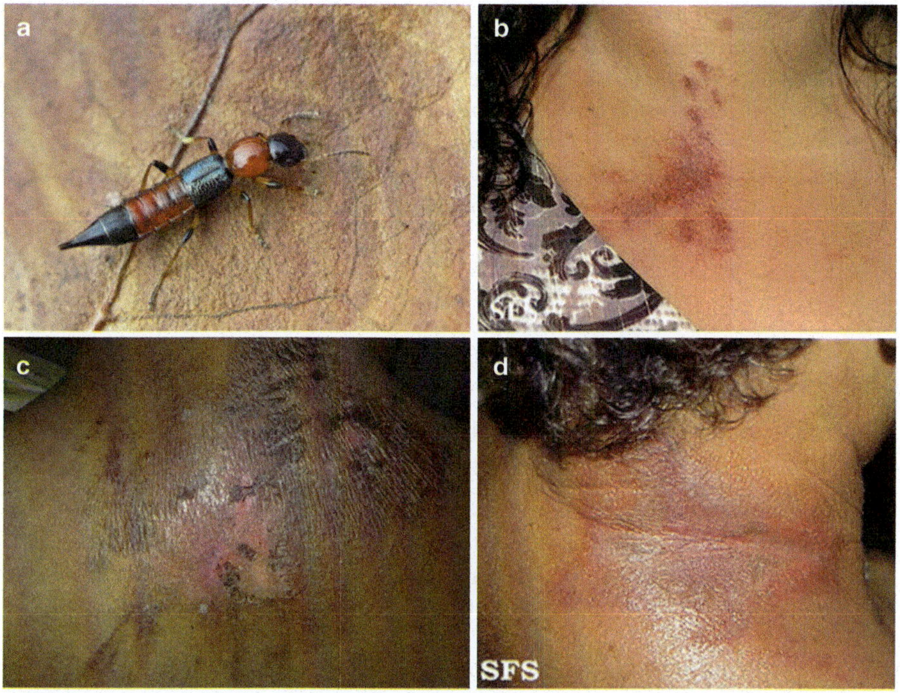

Fig. 14.1 Images of Paederus beetle (**a**) and two patients with Paederus dermatitis skin symptoms. [(**a**) ©Entomart; (**b**, **c**, **d**) ©Samuel Freire da Silva & © Editors, Indian J Dermatol Venereology & Leprology; no change of the images was made]

14.4 Prevention of Paederus Dermatitis

To prevent exposure to *pederin*, the toxic substance from Paederus beetle's body, and prevent the development of Paederus dermatitis, a series of measures can be applied:

- *Avoidance of sitting under artificial light sources*: during seasons of P. dermatitis outbreaks, people in affected areas should avoid to sit close to the sources of fluorescent or incandescent lights.
- *Avoidance of crushing Paederus beetle against the skin*: when the beetle lands on the skin, blow it off instead of crushing it to avoid contact with *pederin.*
- *Closing doors and windows at night:* during the season when the outbreak often occurs, doors and windows can be closed at night to prevent Paederus beetles from getting indoors.
- *Careful use of insecticides*: the use of insecticides can help reduce Paederus beetle population in the living environment; but contamination of the environment by the insecticides should be avoided.

- *Avoidance or removal of vegetation near residential buildings and houses.*
- *Use of light sources that less attract insects (Paederus included), if possible* (Mhalu and Mandara 1981; Taneja et al. 2013; Bong et al. 2013).
- *Washing the body area exposed to pederin with soap to reduce the risk of infection and that of developing the dermatitis.*
- *Clinician consultation should be envisaged, particularly in case of persistence of skin lesions and also in case of periorbital or scrotal involvement* (Vasudevan and Joshi 2010).

14.5 Management of Paederus Dermatitis

After skin contact with Paederus beetle's *pederin*, the following measures can be applied:

- Application of cold wet compresses.
- The use of antihistamine is also advised to reduce the inflammatory response.
- In case of a secondary infection, use an antibiotherapy (oral antibiotics). In the absence of infection, skin lesions generally resolve over time (Cressy et al. 2013; Nasir et al. 2015).
- Some individuals have advised the use of topical corticosteroid on Paederus dermatitis skin lesions; however, healthcare professionals should make sure that the lesions are not infected and that the affected body area is not that large or on the periorbital area. Additionally, except for edematous lesions that often respond to corticosteroids in P. dermatitis, their use on skin wound is generally not recommended (that is also true for P. dermatitis); and a recent study on the experimental model of Paederus dermatitis has shown no clinical benefit of topical dexamethasone (Khaghani et al. 2017).

Considering the elevated number of the victims of Paederus beetle, remedies that can alleviate skin lesions and symptoms and provide better safety profile in Paederus dermatitis management are still needed.

14.6 Conclusion

Paederus dermatitis or dermatitis linearis is a very common condition in several regions of the world, with annual epidemic episodes occurring mostly in tropical zones. The way to prevent the disease outbreaks is to increase awareness among community members and health professionals as well, and implement prophylactic measures such as avoiding to crush the beetle against the skin.

References

Arnold HL, Odam RB, James WD. Parasitic infestations stings and bees. In: Andrew's disease of the skin. 8th ed. Philadelphia: WB Saunders; 1990. p. 486–533.

Banney LA, Wood DJ, Francis GD. Whiplash rove beetle dermatitis in central Queensland. Australas J Dermatol. 2000;41:162–7.

Bazrafkan S, Vtandoost H, Heydari A, et al. Discrimination of Paederus fuscipes and Paederus littoralis by mtDNA-COI PCR-RFLP. J Arthropod Borne Dis. 2016;10(4):454–61.

Beaulieu BA, Irish SR. Literature review of the causes, treatment, and prevention of dermatitis linearis. J Travel Med. 2016;23(4):1–5.

Bong LJ, Kok-Boon N, Jaal Z, et al. Contact toxicity and residual effects of selected insecticides against the adult Paederus fuscipes (Coleoptera: Staphylidae). J Econ Entomol. 2013;106:2530–40.

Cressey BD, Paniz-Mondolfi AE, Rodriguez-Morales AJ, et al. Dermatitis linearis: vesicating dermatosis caused by Paederus species (Coleoptera: Staphylinidae). Case series and review. Wilderness Environ Med. 2013;24(2):124–31.

Frank J, Kanamitsu K. Paederus, sensu lato (Coleoptera: Staphylinidae): natural history and medical importance. J Med Entomol. 1987;24:155–91.

Khaghani R, Mirzaii-Dizgah I, Ghasemi M. Efficacy of Aloe vera cream in the treatment of Paederus dermatitis in mice. J Arthropod Borne Dis. 2017;11(2):204–10.

Lima D, Costa A, Silva F. Abundance and night hourly dispersal of the vesicating beetles of the genus Paederus (Coleoptera: Staphylinidae) attracted to fluorescent, incandescent, and black light sources in the Brazilian savanna. J Med Entomol. 2015;52:50–5.

Mammino JJ. Paederus dermatitis: an outbreak on a medical mission boat in the Amazon. J Clin Aesthet Dermatol. 2011;4(11):44–6.

Markgraf A, Basedow T. Flight activity of predatory Staphylinidae in agriculture in central Germany. J Appl Entomol. 2002;126:79–81.

Maryam S, Fadzly N, Zuharah WF. The effects of light and height of building in attracting Paederus fuscipes Curtis to disperse towards human residential areas. Trop Life Sci Res. 2016;27(1):95–101.

Mhalu FS, Mandara MP. Control of an outbreak of rove beetle dermatitis in an isolated camp in a game reserve. Ann Trop Med Parasitol. 1981;75:231–4.

Nasir S, Akram W, Khan RR, et al. Paederus beetles: the agent of human dermatitis. J Venom Anim Toxins Incl Trop Dis. 2015;21:5.

Penchenier L, Mouchet J, Cros B, et al. Outbreaks of Paederus sabaeus in central Africa: entomological and epidemiological aspects. Bull Soc Pathol Exot. 1994;87:45–8.

Sendur N, Savk E, Karaman G. Paederus dermatitis: a report of 46 cases in Aydin, Turkey. Dermatology. 1999;199(4):353–5.

Sing G, Yousuf Ali S. Paederus dermatitis. Indian J Dermatol Venereol Leprol. 2007;73:13–5.

Sujit SR, Koushik L. Blister beetle dermatitis. Indian J Dermatol Venereol Leprol. 1997;63:69–70.

Taneja A, Sudhir Nayak UK, Shenoi SD. Clinical and epidemiological study of Paederus dermatitis in Manipal, India. J Pak Assoc Dermatol. 2013;23:133–8.

Vasudevan B, Joshi DC. Irritant dermatitis to staphylinid beetle in Indian troops in Congo. Med J Armed Forces India. 2010;66(2):121–4.

Chapter 15
Overview on Other Environmental Skin Disorders

Nlandu Roger Ngatu and Mitsunori Ikeda

Abstract Numerous environmental factors are incriminated in the occurrence of skin disorders. Here, we provide an overview on dermatitis caused by bacteria, Kawasaki disease (KD), and the association between silica-dust exposure and cutaneous autoimmune diseases. Common bacterial skin infections are caused by *Staphylococcus* (S. *aureus*, *S. beta-hemolytic*) and *Streptococcus* (*S. pyogenes*) species, and they include cellulitis, erysipelas, ecthyma, impetigo, and others. On the other hand, folliculitis is caused by a gram-negative bacteria known as *Pseudomonas aeruginosa*. Recently, reports have suggested the infectious origin of KD, and there have been several KD cases reported in Asia and western countries, and KD is considered as a leading cause of acquired heart disease in children population. Recent researchers have discovered KD-specific molecules that share the same structures with microbe-associated molecular patterns (MAMPs), suggesting that KD might have an infectious origin. In the acute phase, KD patients often present with fever, erythema, edema in the extremities and accompanied by pain, exanthema, cervical lymphadenopathy (mostly unilateral, nonsuppurative), conjunctival injection, and changes in the lips and tongue (*strawberry tongue*, a common sign in KD patients) and oropharyngeal mucosa. Occupational silica-dust exposure has been associated with the development of a number of autoimmune diseases, including scleroderma. Additionally, since the work by Erasmus, several case-control studies have demonstrated this association and provided clues on biomarkers (anti-centromeric proteins (anti-CNEP-B in particular), anti-Scl70) that can serve in the early diagnosis of systemic sclerosis or scleroderma as well as a screening tool among silica-dust-exposed workers.

N. R. Ngatu, M.D., Ph.D.
Graduate School of Medicine, International University of Health and Welfare (IUHW), Chiba, Japan

Graduate School of Public Health, International University of Health and Welfare (IUHW), Tokyo, Japan

M. Ikeda, M.D., Ph.D. (✉)
Graduate School of Nursing, and Wellness & Longevity Center, University of Kochi, Kochi, Japan
e-mail: mikeda@cc.u-kochi.ac.jp

N. R. Ngatu, M. Ikeda (eds.), *Occupational and Environmental Skin Disorders*,
https://doi.org/10.1007/978-981-10-8758-5_15

Keywords Cellulitis · Ecthyma · Erysipelas · Folliculitis · Impetigo · Kawasaki disease · Scleroderma

List of Abbreviations

CNEP	Centromeric proteins
KD	Kawasaki disease
Scl	Scleroderma
SSc	Systemic sclerosis

15.1 Brief Introduction

There is a diversity of environmental factors that induce cutaneous disorders. This chapter provides an overview on other skin manifestations and disorders that characterize a number of dermatoses associated with factors that can be found in the work or the living environment, especially diseases of infectious origin (common bacterial skin infections such as cellulitis, erysipelas, folliculitis, impetigo, ecthyma) and cutaneous disorders potentially associated to infectious agents (Kawasaki disease). In addition, highlights on the association between occupational silica-dust exposure and autoimmune diseases, particularly systemic sclerosis/scleroderma, are also provided.

15.2 Cutaneous Bacterial Infections

Numerous infectious agents may be contracted at various occupational or environmental settings. The most common bacterial skin disorders are caused by *Streptococcus* and *Staphylococcus*; they include:

1. *Cellulitis and erysipelas*: both cellulitis and erysipelas are bacterial infections of the skin, with cellulitis extending further deep into the dermis and subcutaneous tissue, mostly the skin of lower limbs, whereas erysipelas involves the upper dermis, mostly on the face. Both infections are clinically characterized by erythema that is often accompanied by lymphangitis and lymphadenopathy. *Streptococcus pyogenes* is the common cause of erysipelas. For cellulitis, *Staphylococcus* (*S. aureus* or *S. beta-hemolytic*) and *Streptococcus* can be the causal agents. The use of antibiotics is the mainstay of treatment (Ibrahim et al. 2015; Sukumaran 2016).
2. *Folliculitis*: it is an inflammation of hair follicle characterized by the presence of pustules in areas of moist skin. The causative agent is *Pseudomonas aeruginosa*. In many cases, Pseudomonas folliculitis occurs a few days after bathing in warm water such as in SPA pool or swimming pool. *Pseudomonas* may resist to common antibiotics against gram-negative bacteria, such as cyclines. An appropriate

and effective antibiotic is advised to manage this disease. Antibiotics of quinolones group (ciprofloxacin, norfloxacin) are often effective.

3. *Impetigo and ecthyma*: impetigo is a contagious cutaneous infection involving the superficial skin caused either by *Streptococcus pyogenes* or *Staphylococcus aureus*. Clinical manifestations include yellowish crusts and sometimes blisters that can be located on the face, the arms, or the legs. Fever is not common in case of impetigo. Currently known risk factors for impetigo include poor nutrition, day care attendance, crowding, contact sports, metabolic disorders such as diabetes, etc. (Hartman-Adams et al. 2014; Ibrahim et al. 2015; Sukumaran 2016). Ecthyma is a non-bullous form of impetigo characterized by sores having fluid or pus inside and erythema. It usually involves the arms and legs; ulcerative lesions and lymphadenopathy can also be seen. The diagnosis is based on skin lesions and symptoms, and both impetigo and ecthyma can be treated with the use of antibiotics (Cole and Gazewood 2007).

15.3 Kawasaki Disease and the Skin

15.3.1 Kawasaki Disease: Definition, Etiology, Epidemiology, and Histopathology

Kawasaki disease (KD) is a systemic vasculitis affecting mostly children under 5 years of age, with a seasonality in some countries. KD consists of an acute febrile condition characterized by an inflammation of arteries of medium size, particularly coronaries, and aneurism. The disease is recognized as a leading cause of acquired heart disease in pediatric population in high-income countries (Newburger et al. 2004; Gupta and Singh 2016).

KD was first reported by Tomisaku Kawasaki, a Japanese pediatrician , in 1960s, and the condition was later on recognized as a new disease by Melish and Hicks in Hawaii in the early 1970s. Similar cases were then reported in different countries, including Greece and Canada in 1975, Australia in 1976, and Germany and Belgium in 1977 (Uehara and Belay 2012). Currently, cases and outbreaks of Kawasaki disease have been reported in more than 60 countries (Asia, Africa, South America, Middle East region, North America, and Europe) (Melish et al. 1976). Korea is reported to be the country with highest KD incidence, reaching 113 per 100,000 children under 5 years of age nationwide in the first decade of the twenty-first century (Park et al. 2011).

Previously, it has been suggested that KD causal agent should be widely distributed in the environment, and no human-to-human contamination could be thought of. Other studies have shown associations between KD and allergy, elevated serum IgE levels, and eosinophilia (Lin and Hwang 1987; Hirao et al. 1987). A decade ago, in a family-based genetic study, Burns et al. (2005) have reported about the association between KD and the genetic variation of IL-4 gene, suggesting that IL-4 plays a role in the pathogenesis of KD. Furthermore, two recent works from Japan have suggested the infectious origin of Kawasaki disease. The first research group found KD-specific molecules that share the same structures with microbe-associated molecular patterns (MAMPs) from *Bacillus cereus*, *Bacillus subtilis*, *Staphylococcus aureus*, and *Yersinia pseudotuberculosis*; they also observed that the serum levels of MAMPs decrease with intravenous immunoglobulin (IVIG) treatment (Kusuda et al. 2014). In addition, Hara (2014) proposed that increased serum levels damage-associated molecular patterns (DAMPs) and MAMPs during the acute phase in KD patients activate the immune system and vascular cells; this leads to release of inflammatory markers such as chemokines and cytokines and induction of KD in genetically predisposed individuals.

The histopathological features include an extensive edema associated with a dilatation of small blood vessels in the papillary dermis. In addition, the cell infiltrates are dominated by mononuclear cells, with a less intense neutrophilic infiltration (Sugawara 1991). Skin biospecimens from Asian KD children showed that cell infiltrates in both the epidermis and the dermis were mainly composed of CD3+ cells and CD14+ macrophages. B cells were not found. This suggests that helper T cells and macrophages might play a crucial role in KD pathogenesis (Sugawara 1991).

15.3.2 Cutaneous Manifestations of Kawasaki Disease

KD is characterized by five major clinical findings occurring in the *acute phase* (10–14 days):

1. Fever, erythema, and edema mostly in the extremities (Fig. 15.1c, d); and they are accompanied by pain.
2. Exanthema (it is generally polymorphous) (Fig. 15.1a).
3. Cervical lymphadenopathy (mostly unilateral and nonsuppurative).
4. Conjunctival injection.
5. Changes in the lips, mouth (tongue in particular), and also oropharyngeal mucosa; "strawberry tongue" is a common sign in KD children (Fig. 15.1b).

Another cutaneous sign consists of the occurrence of erythema or induration at the site of BCG vaccination (Newburger et al. 2004; Gupta and Singh 2016). The cutaneous manifestations that are included in the above list can be crucial in the diagnosis of KD.

The *subacute phase* of KD (2–4 weeks after disease onset) is characterized by a periungual desquamation and resolution of clinical manifestations that were observed in the acute phase, accompanied by elevated markers of inflammation such as C-reactive protein (CRP), erythrocyte sedimentation rate (ESR), and platelet count. Some patients may develop arthritis. In the last phase of KD (convalescent phase), clinical findings and inflammation markers usually return to normal levels.

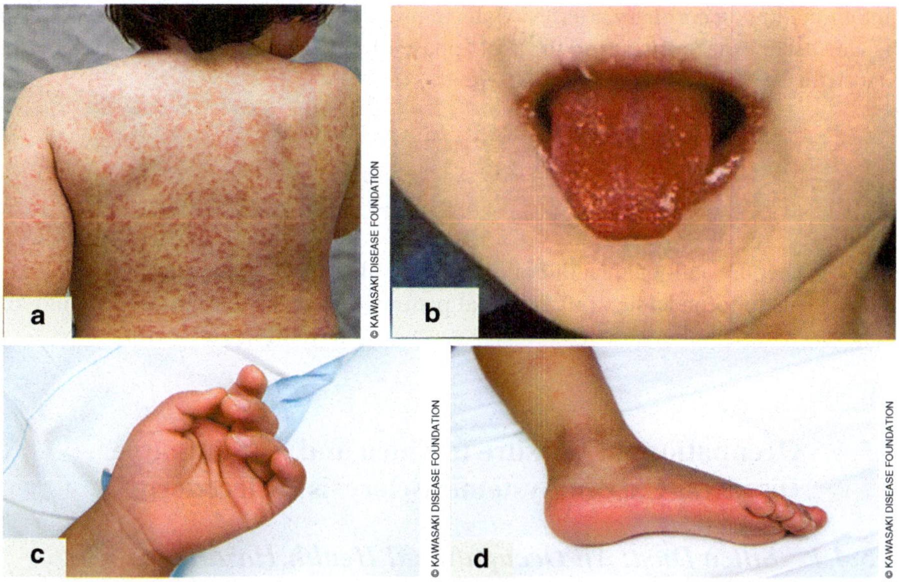

Fig. 15.1 Photos of Kawasaki disease patients showing a skin rash (**a**), strawberry tongue sign (**b**), and erythematous lesions on the upper and lower limbs (extremities) (**c**, **d**) [**a**, **c**, **d**: © Kawasaki Disease Foundation; **b**: Dong S. Kim 2006, ©https://creativecommons.org/licenses/by/4.0/]

For the differential diagnosis of KD, healthcare workers should consider the following pathologies:

- Infectious origin: viruses (herpes viruses, adenovirus, measles, parvovirus), rickettsia (Rocky mountain spotted fever), *Spirocheta* (*Leptospira*), bacteria (*Staphylococcus*, *Streptococcus*)
- Immune reaction (toxic shock syndrome, Stevens-Johnson syndrome)
- Arthritis

In KD patients, non-dermatological clinical findings are numerous; they include radiologic and clinical finings related to the cardiovascular system (abnormal coronary arteries, aneurism, pericarditis, myocarditis, etc.), musculoskeletal system (arthralgia, arthritis), gastrointestinal system (diarrhea, vomiting, abdominal pain, etc.), genitourinary system (pyuria, urethritis), and central nervous system (meningitis, irritability) (Newburger et al. 2004; Park et al. 2011; Gupta and Singh 2016).

15.3.3 Management of Kawasaki Disease

KD patient often recovers well, as the disease is generally self-limited. However, given severe cardiovascular complications that may occur, treatment is needed. Currently, the mainstay of KD treatment is intravenous immunoglobulin to reduce inflammation on coronary arteries' walls in order to reduce thrombosis risk. Aspirin is also used, especially during the acute phase of KD (Singh and Kumar 1996; Kim and Kim 2016; Gupta and Singh 2016).

15.3.4 Conclusion

KD has become a global health issue, affecting almost all regions of the world. It is indispensable to understand its seasonal patterns to get insight into the etiology of this vascular pathology.

15.4 Occupational Exposure to Silica and Autoimmune Diseases: Case of Systemic Sclerosis (Scleroderma)

15.4.1 Silica Dust: An Occupational Health Hazard

Silica or silicon dioxide (SiO2) is an abundant mineral that is quite ubiquitous in the environment, and it is found in rocks, sand, and soil. Silica represents the quarter of the earth's crust; it is also bound to other minerals to form silicates that are used in a number of industries (talc, kaoline, asbestos) (Gamble 1986, Wagner 1997, Ngatu et al. 2012).

Occupational exposure to crystalline silica through inhalation can cause respiratory disorders, mainly silicosis; and silica has been recognized as a carcinogen by the International Agency for Research on Cancer (IARC) (Guha et al. 2011, Ngatu et al. 2012).

15.4.2 Relationship Between Silica and Autoimmune Diseases

Bramwell, a Scottish doctor, was the first to suggest a possible association between occupational silica-dust exposure and autoimmune diseases in 1914. Later on, Erasmus' work that was published in 1957 has attracted the interest of many researchers in the field of industrial health, and, since, many other works conducted examined silica as a possible cause of autoimmune disorders such as systemic sclerosis, rheumatoid arthritis, and systemic lupus erythematosus in Africa, Europe, and North America (Sluis-Cremer et al. 1985, Haustein et al. 1986, Rustin et al. 1990, Parks et al. 1999). In their work, Haustein and colleagues (1990) suggested that, in exposed individuals, crystalline silica less than 5 μm may be phagocytized by macrophages, leading to the release of cytokines and chemokines that activate fibroblasts. This fact will then lead to the increased production of collagen and glycosaminoglycan.

Systemic sclerosis (SSc) is an immune-mediated disease characterized by vasculopathy and fibrosis of the skin and also other organs. The localized form of the disease is called scleroderma (Denton 2017). Several reports have suggested the role played by environmental factors in the occurrence of autoimmune diseases, including SSc (Pollard and Kono 2013; Pollard 2016). Recent animal experiments on silica-induced autoimmune diseases in lupus-prone mice exposed to silica have shown increased levels of markers and conditions associated to autoimmunity such as autoantibodies, high TNF-α levels in the bronchoalveolar fluid (BALF), exacerbation of SLE-like disease, fibrosis, proteinuria, etc. (Bates et al. 2015; Pollard 2015, 2016).

15.4.3 Cutaneous Manifestations and Autoantibodies in Scleroderma Patients and Silica-Exposed Individuals

In the literature, several cases of autoimmune disease in silica-exposed workers are available. Most of those cases were diagnosed during medical screening and treatment for silicosis and others in cohort studies; almost all workers were miners (Cowie 1987, Sanchez-Roman et al. 1993, Parks et al. 1999). Environmental agents that cause scleroderma or systemic sclerosis can be divided in three groups; they comprise those of occupational origin (silica, organic solvents such as vinyl chloride, trichloroethylene, perchloroethylene), agents found in health settings (silicon, silicone implants, bleomycin, L-tryptophan), and other chemicals such as toxic oil (Haustein and Herrmann 1994; Nietert et al. 1998; English et al. 2003; Marie et al. 2014) (Table 15.1).

Common cutaneous manifestations of scleroderma include Raynaud's phenomenon characterized by change in the hand skin color when exposed to cold as the

Table 15.1 Environmental factors/agents associated with scleroderma/systemic sclerosis

Causal agents	Skin symptoms/disorders
1. Occupational exposure:	
– *Organic solvents (Vinyl chloride, tricholoroethylene, perchloroethylene)* – *Silica, welding fume*	– Sclerodactyly, plaque-like fibrotic cutaneous lesions, Raynaud's phenomenon – Systemic sclerosis/scleroderma (Haustein and Herrmann 1994; Nietert et al. 1998; English et al. 2003, Marie et al. 2014)
2. Iatrogenic factors and others:	
– *Pentazocine* – *Bleomycin* – l-*Tryptophan* – *Silicone implants* – *Toxic oil*	– Sclerotic fibrosis on the injection sites, skin ulceration, changes in pigmentation – Scleroderma-like skin lesions – Sclerodermatous skin induration, arthralgia – Systemic sclerosis/scleroderma, Sjogren's syndrome, arthritis Scleroderma-like changes, neuromuscular atrophy (English et al. 2003, Marie et al. 2014)

main clinical feature; other symptoms are pruritus, telangiectasia, morphea, alternation of hypo- and hyperpigmentation on the limbs (the salt and pepper appearance), tightening of the skin, and skin ulcer (Adnan 2008; Toledano et al. 2009).

Serum autoantibody levels have a clinical relevance and play an important role in the diagnosis and the prognosis of autoimmune disorders, and centromeric proteins (CENP-A and CENP-B), anti-keratinocyte antibodies (AKA), and anti-Scl70 have been extensively investigated. A study conducted in Indian scleroderma patients (all in acute phase of disease) showed high level of anti-Scl70, anti-centromere, anti-endothelial cell antibodies (AECA), and anti-keratinocyte antibodies (AKA) in scleroderma patients with diffused cutaneous SSc compared to those with limited cutaneous SSc (Volpe et al. 2009; Pradhan et al. 2014).

A study on markers of autoimmunity in sera from uranium miners has suggested that CENP-B could serve as target marker for the diagnosis of autoimmune diseases in silica-exposed individuals (Conrad et al. 1995). Additionally, other recent studies on the relationship between silica, silicosis, and autoimmune diseases have focused on Scl-70, ANA, ANCA, rheumatoid factor (RF), and centromeric proteins (CENP-A and CENP-B). Zaghi et al. (2010) found that RF was associated with silicosis, whereas the other levels of other markers were not that high in those patients. More recently, a study showed that, of the markers studied in silicotic patients, only anti-CENP-B was positively associated with silicosis (Lee et al. 2017), suggesting that anti-CENP-B might be an important marker in the early diagnosis of autoimmunity in individuals with occupational or environmental exposure to silica. The abovementioned research findings suggest the usefulness of anti-CENP as candidate marker with high potential to serve in screening and early diagnosis of autoimmune disorders in silica-exposed individuals.

References

Bates MA, Brandnberger C, Langohr I, et al. Silica triggers inflammation and ectopic lymphoid neogenesis in the lungs in parallel with accelerated onset of systemic autoimmunity and glomerulonephritis in the lupus-prone NZBWFI mouse. PLoS One. 2015;10:e125481.

Burns JC, Shimizu C, Shike H, et al. Family-based association analysis implicated IL-4 in susceptibility to Kawasaki disease. Genes Immun. 2005;6(5):438–44.

Cole C, Gazewood J. Diagnosis and treatment of impetigo. Am Fam Physician. 2007;75(6):859–64.

Conrad K, Stahnke G, Liedvogel B, et al. Anti-CENP-B response in sera of uranium miners exposed to quartz dust and patients with possible development of systemic sclerosis (scleroderma). J Rheumatol. 1995;22(7):1286–94.

Cowie RL. Silica-dust-exposed mine workers with scleroderma (systemic sclerosis). Chest. 1987;92(2):260–2.

Denton CP. Systemic sclerosis. Lancet. 2017;390(10103):1685–99.

Adnan ZA. Diagnosis and treatment of scleroderma. Acta Med Indones. 2008;40(2):109–12.

English JSC, Dawe RS, Ferguson J. Environmental effects and skin disease. Br Med Bull. 2003;68:129–42.

Pollard KM. Environment, autoantibodies, and autoimmunity. Front Immunol. 2015;6:60.

Gamble JF. Silicate pneumoconiosis. In: Merchant JA, editor. Occupational respiratory diseases. Washington, DC: Government Printing Office; 1986. p. p243. Publication No. DHHS (NIOSH) 86-102.
Guha N, Straif K, Benbrahim-Tallaa L. The IARC monograph on the carcinogenicity of crystalline silica. Med Lav. 2011;102(4):310–20.
Gupta A, Singh S. Kawasaki disease for dermatologists. Indian Dermatol Online J. 2016;7(6):461–70.
Hara T. Kawasaki disease and innate immunity. Nihon Rinsho. 2014;72:1542–7.
Hartman-Adams H, Banvard C, Juckett G. Impetigo: diagnosis and treatment. Am Fam Physician. 2014;90(4):229–35.
Haustein UF, Herrmann K. Environmental scleroderma. Clin Dermatol. 1994;12(3):467–73.
Haustein UF, Herrmann K, Bohmf HJ. Pathogenesis of progressive systemic sclerosis. Int J Dermatol. 1986;25(5):286–94.
Haustin UF, Ziegler V, Hermann K, et al. Silica-induced scleroderma. J Am Acad Dermatol. 1990;22:444–8.
Hirao J, Yoshimura N, Homma N, et al. Immunological studies on Kawasaki disease: II. Isolation and characterization of an immunosuppressive factor in acute phase sera. Clin Exp Immunol. 1987;67:433–40.
Ibrahim F, Khan T, Pujalte GG. Bacterial skin infections. Prim Care. 2015;42(4):485–99.
Kim KY, Kim DS. Recent advances in Kawasaki disease. Yonsei Med J. 2016;57(1):15–21.
Kusuda T, Nakashima Y, Kanno S, et al. Kawasaki disease-specific molecules in the sera are linked to microbe-associated molecular patterns in the biofilms. PLoS One. 2014;9:e113054.
Lee S, Hayashi H, Kumagai-Takei N, et al. Clinical evaluation of CENP-B and Scl70 autoantibodies in silicosis patients. Exp Ther Med. 2017;13:2616–22.
Lin CY, Hwang B. Serial immunologic studies in patients with mucocutaneous lymph node syndrome (Kawasaki disease). Ann Allergy. 1987;59:291–7.
Marie I, Gehanno JF, Bubenheim M, et al. Prospective study to evaluate the association between systemic sclerosis and occupational exposure and review of the literature. Autoimmun Rev. 2014;13(2):151–6.
Melish ME, Hicks RM, Larson E. Mucocutaneous lymph node syndrome in the United States. Am J Dis Child. 1976;130:599–607.
Newburger JW, Takahasi M, Gerber MA, et al. Diagnosis, treatment and long-term management of Kawasaki disease: a statement for health professionals from the Committee on Rheumatic Fever, Endocarditis and Kawasaki Disease, Council on Cardiovascular Disease in the Young, American Heart Association. Circulation. 2004;110:2747–71.
Ngatu NR, Kayembe NJM, Longo-Mbenza B et al. The Pneumoconioses. In: Elvisegran Malcolm Irusen, editor. Lung diseases-selected state of the art reviews. Intech; 2012. ISBN: 978-953-51-0180-2. http://www.intechopen.com/books/lungdiseases-selected-state-of-the-art-reviews/the-pneumoconioses.
Nietert PJ, Sytherland SE, Silver RM, et al. Is occupational organic solvent exposure a risk factor for scleroderma? Arthritis Rheum. 1998;41(6):1111–8.
Park YW, Han JW, Hong YM, et al. Epidemiologic features of Kawasaki disease in Korea, 2006–2008. Pediatr Int. 2011;53:36–9.
Parks CG, Conrad K, Cooper GS. Occupational exposure to crystalline silica and autoimmune disease. Environ Health Perspect. 1999;107(5):793–8.
Pollard KM, Kono DH. Requirements for innate immune pathways in environmentally induced autoimmunity. BMC Med. 2013;11:100.
Pradhan V, Rajadhyaksha A, Nadkar M, et al. Clinical and autoimmune profile of scleroderma patients from western India. Int J Rheumatol. 2014;2014:983781.
Rustin MH, Bull HA, Ziegler V, et al. Silica-associated systemic sclerosis is clinically, serologically and immunologically indistinguishable from idiopathic systemic sclerosis. Br J Dermatol. 1990;123:725–34.

Sanchez-Roman J, Wichmann I, Salaberri J, et al. Multiple clinical and biological autoimmune manifestations in 50 workers after occupational exposure to silica. Ann Rheum Dis. 1993;52(7):534–8.

Pollard KM. Silica, silicosis, and autoimmunity. Front Immunol. 2016;7:97.

Singh S, Kumar L. Kawasaki disease: treatment with intravenous immunoglobulin during the acute stage. Indian Pediatr. 1996;33:689–92.

Sluis-Cremer GK, Hessel PA, Nizdo EH, et al. Silica, silicosis, and progressive systemic sclerosis. Br J Ind Med. 1985;42:838–43.

Sugawara T. Immunopathology of skin lesions in Kawasaki disease (published in japanese). Arerugi 1991;40(4):476–82.

Sukumaran V. Bacterial skin and soft tissue infections. Aust Prescr. 2016;39(5):159–63.

Toledano C, Rabhi S, Kettaneh A, et al. Localized scleroderma: a series of 52 patients. Eur J Intern Med. 2009;20(3):331–6.

Uehara R, Belay ED. Epidemiology of Kawasaki disease in Asia, Europe, and the United States. J Epidemiol. 2012;22(2):79–85.

Volpe A, Ruzzenente O, Caramaschi P, et al. Clinical associations of anti-CENP-B and anti-Scl70 antibody levels measured by multiplexed fluorescent microsphere immunoassay in systemic sclerosis. Rheumatol Int. 2009;29(9):1073–9.

Wagner GR. Asbestosis and silicosis. Lancet. 1997;349:1311.

Zaghi G, Koga F, Nisihara RM, et al. Autoantibodies in silicosis patients and silica-exposed individuals. Rheumatol Int. 2010;30(8):1071–5.

The manufacturer's authorised representative in the EU is Springer Nature Customer Service Centre GmbH, Europaplatz 3, 69115 Heidelberg, Germany. If you have any concerns regarding our products, please contact ProductSafety@springernature.com

Printed and bound by CPI Group (UK) Ltd, Croydon, CR0 4YY

25/09/2026

02222845-0004